I've Been Diagnosed, Now What?

Courageously Fighting Cancer in the Face of Fear,
Uncertainty and Doubt

Katrece Nolen

NMG Publishing

First edition 2020

ISBN 978-1-7352250-0-5 (Paperback)
ISBN 978-1-7352250-1-2 (eBook)

This book is not intended as a substitute for the medical advice of physicians. The reader should regularly consult a physician in matters relating to his/her health, particularly with respect to any symptoms that may require diagnosis or medical attention.

For my husband, Keith, and our children, Kelci, Kendall, and Keith Jr.
You are my world.

Table of Contents

Preface

I received the first ideas for writing this book in the fall of 2016. I had been struggling with what would be next in my life. It had been three years since I had come home from the hospital after having surgery in my fight against cancer.

It had been a long three years of surviving the shock of what my family and I had gone through during almost a year of active cancer treatment and the mental games one goes through following treatment.

Holding off the fears of recurrence with every checkup can be unnerving, but at the three-year mark, I decided it was time to let go of the fear of figuring out how to survive. I would get beyond survival.

How was I going to do that, what would it look like, and what would it mean? To answer these questions, I had to take the focus off ME. I needed to start focusing on how I could help others get beyond survival mode and learn how to flourish, regardless of their stage of cancer treatment.

I reflected and considered the things that helped me get the best treatment and support possible while undergoing treatment. The way I did it was through research, asking lots of questions, and learning from others in my cancer network.

Through these actions and my desire to live, I learned how to build a superior medical team and surround myself with an excellent support team of family and friends who were available to me both in-person and remotely.

Most times, I learned about options for treatment for the type of cancer I had from private communities on social media. Often, I would think about those who might not be as resourceful as me. Perhaps they had the financial means but felt isolated from family or friends. Maybe they were not computer savvy enough to conduct research. It triggered a desire in me to teach other survivors how they, their family members, and friends can build support communities to help them through this period of their lives.

In this book, I will share my own experiences and real-life experiences from other cancer survivors. In their own words, they will share how they found the best support.

I hope that sharing these experiences will not only give you insight into the available support options but the strength and courage to face your cancer journey. I hope this book moves you from an attitude of surviving to one of living a life beyond survival.

Ultimately, I want you to know that you need not go through this alone. Help is out there and available for you. Don't give up!

Introduction

I remember it like it was yesterday. It had been less than six months since I'd completed my cancer treatments. I was glad the heavy lifting was over, and I was settling into my new "normal."

Earlier that week, we ran into one of my husband's buddies and found out he was undergoing treatment for his second cancer diagnosis. Later that same week, we visited his family, and I began asking questions. I often did this with families I met who were undergoing cancer treatment. I wanted to understand how they were handling treatment and how they felt about the nearby cancer support center.

To my surprise, they had never heard about the center. Their response left me reeling. This family was going through a second cancer diagnosis, and their local oncologist hadn't shared this wealth of cancer support services. A local center right around the corner from their home offered free, specialized support services, and they had not been made aware of its existence. How could this be? I then wondered how many other families fighting cancer were in a similar situation?

Because I was curious, I began doing some research on finding support. I found some troubling statistics in a report issued by the Cancer Support community,[1] which stated that "More than half of respondents

---

1   "Access to Care in Cancer: Barriers and Challenges | Cancer Community" n.d.

reported not receiving social and/or emotional support as part of their cancer care. Nearly 70% of those reported that they would have liked to have received such services. A quarter (25%) of those surveyed did not feel confident they received the care that they needed."

Reading these troubling statistics got me thinking about my cancer journey and how devastated I was following my diagnosis to learn about the low survival rates. Someone in my cancer support group told me we shouldn't pay attention to those statistics because it was an average, and everyone responds differently to treatment, has different circumstances and varying levels of access to care.

Such a large percentage of patients felt they were not receiving the social and emotional support services they so desperately needed. I understood why cancer treatment outcomes varied. This knowledge increased my desire to understand why these services were not made available or communicated to all cancer patients.

I began by revisiting my story. I was misdiagnosed and nearly turned away when attempting to get the proper diagnosis due to "paperwork issues." Yet, I stood my ground and got access to the medical services I needed. I believe the only reason I got through this trying period in my life was because of my self-advocacy, learning about the plethora of support and resources that surrounded me.

I wondered what would happen if more patients and caregivers felt empowered to become their own best advocates? Would more people survive this deadly disease and live a longer life?

Thousands of organizations exist to provide valuable information and cancer support. This information ranges from specifics about cancer types to the treatments available to combat the disease. So, why do so many survivors think that they do not receive the help they need?

Think about it – a cancer diagnosis is not a regular occurrence like getting a common cold or an ear infection. After you have had a few colds or ear infections, you recognize the symptoms, get treatment, and recover. For someone diagnosed with cancer, they have not been conditioned to figure out what to do. It's such a steep learning curve to find help in a condensed period. Most patients don't know what resources exist.

If I were to identify the one place every cancer patient can at least attempt to find help, it would be the oncology office. It should be the first line of support. Some oncology practices are rightfully focused on treating the disease but may miss the mark on the social and emotional support a cancer survivor needs.

I would like to see policies instituted to refer all patients to mental health services. Such a plan could help address patients who don't want to ask for help because they believe it's a sign of weakness or a loss of control over their circumstances. Who wants to give up control over their life?

For example, I was exhausted following my first cancer treatment, but I still tried to cook and clean for my family of five. I wanted to maintain as much normalcy as possible.

I fondly remember my Mom staying with our family a few times during my cancer treatment. Even with her present, I tried to stick to all my usual routines.

Mom confronted me and asked why I was trying to do all these things, waving off any offers of support when she was specifically there to help my family and me out.

She told me to stop trying to be a superwoman and focus on healing. She instructed me to let others help with everything else. I was taking away their joy of helping our family get through this period of our lives.

Years later, I read a blog post by Mike Robbins, titled, "It's OK to Ask for Help"[2] and how we "get a little funny asking for help." He states how under normal circumstances, it's hard for people to ask for help from others, but it's also ironic that many of us love to help others.

Why the imbalance? We must give ourselves permission to ask for and accept help. We must be confident and not fear a negative response when asking for help. Mike Robbins suggests that genuine requests for support be made without being so tightly attached to a positive or negative response. In other words, don't think the world will end if the answer is "No." He also suggests that we need to accept support, be thankful for any support offered, and let them respond to the request in their unique way.

Sometimes, a person may be incapable of asking for help. They may be mentally or physically unable to request the specific support that they need. In these cases, you must rely upon a network of doctors, cancer patient navigators, family members, and friends. Begin by admitting your limitations and asking others to help fill the gap. Hold the conversation as soon as possible after the diagnosis.

Assume you will need help and identify the circle of support that can assist when needed. This book can help fill the gap for people who are struggling with what questions to ask or understanding the resources available.

You'll see survivor secrets throughout the book that can help you create a customized cancer support plan. A recent study by MedScape[3] reports that "It's when they (patients) go back home that all the questions arise, so the key message for me there is [this]: put in place ancillary services, for example, specialist cancer nurses, nurse navigators or cancer navigators...who can play the companion role for patients and their families and answer questions in between those doctor visits."

2   m.huffpost.com/us/entry/814796
3   Cancer Patients Report Lack of Info and Support

In this book, you won't find all the answers, but I will try my best to guide you on how to find the tools and resources to make better choices regarding your support. The answer is not just about fighting the disease, but it's also about surrounding survivors and families with the support they need to give them hope and the perseverance to sustain the fight.

I share aspects of the journey through my personal story and those of others because two different approaches to solving the issue at hand can cause similar or differing outcomes.

The book highlights available resources and provides insights, survivor secrets, and guidance on a myriad of approaches that cancer survivors, family members, and caregivers can take to gain access to needed support functions and services. It spans the periods of my cancer diagnosis, treatment, and return to normalcy.

Please know the steps of your journey might occur in a different sequence, but I hope this book will help to improve positive outcomes for everyone who reads it.

Part 1

MY LIFE CHANGED

CHAPTER 1:
Something's Different

From the onset, I knew something was wrong. I honestly believe that playing with my 3-year-old son on the family room floor saved my life. It was just after the new year towards the end of January and nearing my 38th birthday. I was crawling on the floor and chasing after my son when I looked down inside the collar of my t-shirt and noticed that one breast looked slightly bigger than the other. I ignored it for a little while but looked down a few minutes later and thought there was a difference in the size of my breasts. This time, I asked my husband if he noticed a difference, but he said they looked the same.

Later that night, I stood alone, naked in front of our bathroom mirror, and stared at the same breast, which now definitely appeared swollen. I was convinced there was a difference and again asked my husband if he noticed a difference. This time, he answered yes.

It was so noticeable I placed a call to the office of my family doctor first thing the next morning. My regular family doctor was not in the office that day, and they asked if I wanted to wait until she returned the next day. I told them this couldn't wait another day, so I would see any doctor available in the medical practice.

They could get me in for an appointment that afternoon with a male doctor. I was a bit reluctant to visit with a male doctor concerning my breasts and would have preferred a female physician, but something told me I needed to be seen rather quickly.

During the examination, the doctor asked me a few specific questions: how long had it been since I noticed this change, and how long had it been since I had nursed our son? I told him the swelling was first noticeable the day before and had become more pronounced in a matter of hours. It had been nearly 2.5 years since I nursed our 3-year-old son as I had only nursed him for three months.

The doctor conducted a physical examination of my breasts and commented that the left breast, which was noticeably bigger, felt warm to the touch. He indicated the swelling might be caused by an infection typically seen in nursing mothers called mastitis, but since it had been such a long time since I last nursed my child, such a diagnosis would be out of the ordinary.

He said he would prescribe an antibiotic, but for cautionary reasons, he wanted me to schedule a mammogram as soon as possible. On my behalf, they contacted the facility directly to schedule the mammogram for the following morning.

He told me one thing I very much appreciate to this day. Because of this unusual circumstance, even if the results of the mammogram came back normal, I should follow up with a breast specialist to establish a baseline for my breast health and seek continuous monitoring from their practice. He handed me a card for a local breast specialist he considered to be one of the best in our immediate area. Later, that card would become very handy.

CHAPTER 2:

My Very First Mammogram

The next morning, I checked into a local radiology center to undergo my very first mammogram. They fit me right in, and after changing my clothes, I went into the back, where a lovely mammography technician led me to a machine. She helped me place my non-swollen breast onto the mammography slide and pressed down on the breast tissue. It wasn't comfortable.

She then did the same thing with the swollen breast. It was so excruciatingly painful it brought tears to my eyes. I remember the technician apologizing profusely for having to put me through such pain. After that, I went into another room where they performed an ultrasound of the breasts. After completing these examinations, I got dressed and was directed to a separate area to await my results.

A radiologist visited with me in the private waiting area and informed me they could not detect any lumps or mass in my breast tissue and that the dense tissue found in the swollen breast was because of mastitis. They recommended I continue to take the antibiotic to get rid of the infection. I left, relieved it was not something more serious.

I continued taking the antibiotics for the prescribed period, but I found that instead of the swelling going down, it had increased. My breast was so swollen I could no longer button my blouse. I was worried before, but now, I was panicking. I recalled my family practice doctor recommending that even if the mammogram came back normal, I should schedule an appointment with a breast surgeon and have them monitor my breasts. Thankfully, I kept the business card he gave me and contacted their office to schedule an appointment right away.

The weirdest thing happened when I called to schedule the appointment. I was told there was at least a one- to two-month wait. I expressed the urgency of the situation and the need to be scheduled as quickly as possible but was told there was nothing they could do.

That answer was not good enough for me. I pressed to be seen by another breast surgeon in their office. Another surgeon was available, and they scheduled an appointment for later in the week. I was surprised an offer to meet with another doctor at the practice was not readily made.

The appointment scheduler requested I bring the results from the mammography to this appointment. I knew it would be no problem because I already had the results provided to me on a CD-ROM.

During the appointment check-in, the receptionist asked me for the medical records, and I handed over the CD-ROM. After a few minutes, the receptionist called me back to the check-in desk and indicated that unless they received the actual mammography film and not the CD-ROM, the visit would have to be rescheduled. What did this lady just say to me? Was she serious?

I did not remember the request to provide a mammography film and asked if I could proceed with my appointment. At the very least, I wanted an opportunity to consult with the doctor about my symptoms and have the film sent over the following business day. The receptionist indicated the appointment could not proceed without the film.

I thought it utterly ridiculous to be turned away without at least seeing the surgeon, so I asked to meet with the office manager. During this entire time, I was conversing with my husband over the phone, telling him how I felt I was being treated, and he said he was on his way.

The office manager called me back to her workspace and again apologized that I could not proceed with my scheduled appointment. In any other situation, I would have probably walked out of the office to find another doctor. Instead, I remained sitting in the manager's office, pleading my case, and refusing to leave without being seen by the surgeon.

Lo-and-behold, after a few minutes of back and forth with the office manager, the surgeon came into the manager's office, introduced herself, and was apologetic about being unable to see me that day. She explained the need to have all the information at her fingertips to provide a diagnosis. The CD-ROM was not enough because their practice did not have the monitors on-site that would give them the ability to review the results from the mammogram image on the CD-ROM.

The monitors in their practice did not have the correct pixel capacity to review the picture in detail. As a result, their office had to use the mammography film to detect any abnormalities. She pointed to a file folder she held in her hands and indicated she had been reviewing my case.

The surgeon explained in briefly reading about my symptoms and knowing how long it had been since I'd first reported symptoms and seeing me in person, she suspected I had Inflammatory Breast Cancer.

Yes, you heard it right. I was sitting next to a desk in the manager's office, not in the exam room when I learned I might have Inflammatory Breast Cancer.

In my head, I'm thinking, "Wait, what?!" For the last 30 minutes, I have been fighting to get back here to see you, even offering to pay out-of-pocket, so they would see me. Instead, I was told a missing mammography film would prevent me from being seen that day, and I needed to reschedule for another day.

Oh, my word, I was hot! She could come to this preliminary conclusion without the film, so why put me through this madness?! But get this – later, I learned most cases of Inflammatory Breast Cancer (IBC) are NOT DETECTABLE with a mammogram or ultrasound! So, all this hoopla about the mammogram was just that – HOOPLA! There was no reason the doctor couldn't take the time to at least continue with a consultation without the mammogram film. The time was blocked, and I was a customer willing to pay out of pocket.

The surgeon explained that she would need to perform a skin biopsy because IBC presents itself in the skin tissue of the breast. The biopsy would be a quick way to verify cancer. She asked if she could perform the biopsy the following morning (as the office was now closed), and she would then send it to pathology for testing and ask them to rush the results.

She asked if I was okay, and I said I would have to be, and I was just glad to get moving on this thing. She told me my husband was waiting to see me out near the reception area. She met him on her way to the office manager's room and wanted to assure him she was heading to see me. That's what I call Team Nolen! I returned to the receptionist to schedule the skin biopsy for the following morning.

Survivor Secret: How to Prepare for Your First Breast Surgeon Visit

- **When Scheduling the Appointment:** Ask the scheduler to provide you with a link to the new patient registration portal on their website or to email a copy of a document detailing all of the required information you should submit before the appointment.

- **If you have had a mammogram and prior breast exams** conducted by your family doctor, then obtain a copy of the doctor's notes, reports and imaging. Check with the office of the breast surgeon to verify how they would like to receive any prior imaging reports. Specifically ask if they need to have the film or if the CD or DVD image will be sufficient.

- **If your 1st choice doctor is not available** to schedule an appointment within a 2-week period, check to see if there are other surgeons in the practice who can meet with you. If they are not available, ask for a referral to another doctor. If they are unable to refer you to a doctor, ask your family doctor or OB-GYN for another referral.

- If you check into your surgeon's office and have **difficulty proceeding with your scheduled appointment**, ask to speak with the office manager and ask to go to their office for a private conversation. Explain your situation and see if they can get you back to see the doctor.

CHAPTER 3:
Waiting for Answers

I had NEVER heard of Inflammatory Breast Cancer (IBC). Heck, I didn't even know there were DIFFERENT types of breast cancer. I did what any information seeker would do; I left the surgeon's office, drove to our nearest grocery store (because I still had grocery shopping to do), and looked up Inflammatory Breast Cancer in Google Search.

I did NOT like the Google search results. I was in the grocery store parking lot reading about IBC when I burst into tears. I learned IBC is one of the most aggressive forms of breast cancer. The earliest state of detection was Stage 3. It is rare, and the chances of survival from this form of breast cancer is low. With this heaviness in my heart, I pulled myself together, went grocery shopping, and went home to a typical evening with the family. That night, my husband and I spoke about our faith and how we were confident we would get through this thing together.

They performed the skin biopsy the next morning, and it was uneventful. The appointment was on a Friday, and the surgeon indicated she would request a rush on the evaluation. The results could be in as early as Monday or Tuesday evening. Thankfully, she wouldn't make me come back into the office to find out the results but would call me to share the news and relay the next steps.

That was one LONG weekend. I cried a few times, and we called my parents to let them know what was going on. They were shocked at what was happening and said they would be there for us, regardless of the results, and were praying for the best outcome.

About mid-afternoon on that following Monday, my cell phone rang. I looked at the caller ID and saw it was the breast surgeon's office. My heart pounded as I answered the call. The surgeon said the results had come back positive for cancer and would like to meet with me the following day. I thanked her for calling me and hung up the phone. I didn't cry then because I think I was all cried out from the weekend and perhaps still a bit in shock.

I called my husband to tell him the news. He assured me that we could fight this. I was so shocked, the only thing I could think of to do next was to make a crab boil for dinner. After I got home, I tried to cook the crab but soon discovered my cooking pot was not big enough for the crab legs. Did I give up? Nope, I asked my husband to take me to the department store that evening to purchase a brand new, extra-large cooking pot. I went into the store while my husband waited outside in the van with our kids.

At the checkout counter, I saw my church pastor's wife. I had NEVER seen her out shopping before. She saw me, came over, and asked me how I was doing. I told her I wasn't doing so well. I was buying this new pot to cook in, but I had just learned I had cancer that afternoon. She was shocked at the news but quickly assured me it would be all right, and that she and our pastor would pray for me.

I couldn't believe I would have a chance encounter like that on a school night. I am a woman of faith, and seeing the pastor's wife at that moment meant the world to me. It gave me a sense of calm that everything would be all right. I went home with my brand-new pot and a touch of HOPE and made a delicious crab boil.

My Mom and Dad were a significant part of my care support team from just after finding out that I had cancer until this present day. Here are words shared by my Mom on how she felt at the very beginning of the journey.

"*I remember being told our daughter had an appointment with the doctor because she was concerned about her breast being swollen. Later, she shared the doctor said she had cancer. That dreaded word was ringing in my head. Just thinking about it now and reliving that moment makes my heart beat faster.*

I thought, "Cancer, oh no, not my baby!" Thinking about that time brings tears to my eyes. Not my baby! God, no!!!! Don't let this happen to my baby. I was in a daze. I could not believe this was happening to our family.... our daughter.

That night, my husband held me close to him, comforting me while dealing with his emotional pain, trying to remain strong.

I thought, "Oh, God. No, please tell me that this is not true." I cried myself to sleep, trying not to disturb my husband as he laid next to me in bed, dealing with this word cancer that now affected our family.

I remember asking God to please not take our daughter away from her family and us as they needed her. Keith needed her, and the kids needed her. I cried again, just thinking about what would happen to our family without her, especially with her kids being so young and the youngest being only three years old.

We prayed and prayed and prayed some more, asking God to watch over our daughter, her family, and the rest of the family as we started on the journey that was so unknown to us.

We told our daughter we would be there for her and the family as we fought this dreaded disease together! We told our daughter we would take time off from work to be there with her during treatment."

CHAPTER 4:

I'm Not Qualified to Select a Cancer Team!

The doctor told me I would need to select a team of cancer doctors to fight the disease. I felt anxious because HOW IN THE WORLD WAS I QUALIFIED to choose my team of cancer doctors who would be responsible for getting rid of the cancer growing inside of me, so I wouldn't DIE?!

It seemed to be such a big decision for me to make, but looking back, I can understand why they wanted it to be MY decision. I just wish there had been a little more support available in making this critical decision. Instead, my doctor sat in front of me at a long table and laid out a series of business cards. She explained that based upon the cancer diagnosis, I would need to have a breast surgeon, a hematology oncologist for chemotherapy treatment, a radiation oncologist for radiation treatments, and a plastic surgeon for breast reconstruction.

Next, she laid out a series of business cards representing doctors with various specialties. Pointing at each business card, she explained each doctor's specialty and her opinion of their level of patient engagement. She assessed their level of patient engagement or bedside manner on their willingness to answer questions and how well they explained treatment plans in layman's terms. She summarized the feedback she had received from her patients over the years.

From these brief explanations, at the end of this 30-minute discussion, I made a preliminary decision on the members of my cancer team. The doctor instructed me to call each one of them to schedule an introductory appointment, with the priority to call the hematology oncologist, otherwise known as the Chemo Doctor, because the first treatment would begin with this doctor.

She requested that following our discussion, I should meet with a nursing assistant in her practice, who would help me with scheduling the diagnostic testing.

The nursing assistant worked with me to schedule a biopsy to verify the cancer type. She told me the hospital had nurse navigators who were a valuable resource and suggested I reach out to them. I asked her about scheduling the rest of the appointments with the other cancer doctors, and she told me that would be something I should complete myself because I knew the specifics of my schedule.

In the discussion with the doctor, she said it was important to schedule the chemo doctor first, the radiation oncologist next, and finally, the plastic surgeon. Treatment would begin with chemotherapy, followed by surgery, radiation, and, eventually, plastic surgery. I left the office still worried about my situation, but pleased I had a specific set of next steps that would get me closer to treatment.

What stuck in my mind was IBC as an aggressive form of cancer. My biggest priority was scheduling those additional appointments as soon as possible. I feared that if I did not get these appointments scheduled quickly and begin treatment, I would be at risk of the cancer spreading and maybe progressing to Stage 4.

It wasn't tough to contact the medical offices to request an appointment. The only hurdle was convincing them that my appointment needed to be scheduled sooner rather than later because I potentially had an aggressive form of cancer.

WAITING for the tests and the results was excruciating. In my mind, I should have been fast-tracked for all my appointments. Instead, it was nearly two weeks before I completed all my doctor visits and diagnostics testing.

Case in point, I went to one diagnostic center for a procedure called a punch biopsy. Yep, it was just as painful as it sounds. They took a device shaped like a gun and aimed it at my breast. They pulled the trigger, and it immediately punched a hole in my breast and extracted breast tissue to biopsy. Thankfully, they numbed the area before the test, but it was still scary.

The doctor who observed the technician perform the test procedure asked me when I was scheduled for my breast MRI. I told her I was not planned for one and asked if I should be concerned. She said that usually, they scheduled the breast MRI to take place right after the punch biopsy as it helps in determining the type of cancer.

Besides extracting tissue to type the cancer, the tool used for the punch biopsy also serves as a method of inserting a marker in the breast tissue to assist with further tests. Following up with a breast MRI creates a 3-D picture of the breast with the location of the marker serving as a kind of anchor point to baseline and track the potential spread of the cancer.

After hearing this explanation, I got upset, even shedding tears. I wondered if it was standard practice to schedule these tests back to back. Knowing the difficulty in planning this diagnostic test, why in the world would the doctor not order the breast MRI and instead, wait for me to return with the results of the punch biopsy and then send me back to this same location for the breast MRI?

My goodness - I just kept thinking this thing was aggressive, and I didn't have much time to clown around with the surgeon who sent me here for inadequate testing. I felt the surgeon was NOT doing her job correctly, and I was not only upset but pissed.

The doctor at the biopsy told me not to worry about it. They would check availability and make the arrangements to have me complete the breast MRI as soon as a slot opened for that day. She contacted my breast surgeon to get the orders. While we waited for the doctor, the nurse who assisted with the punch biopsy, saw how distressed I was upon hearing the news about the need for a second test. She comforted me and told me everything would be all right. She even prayed with me on the spot.

The doctor returned with wonderful news. They could fit me in for the breast MRI within the next few hours. I was thankful for the news, and the time it would save. Still, I kept thinking about how it would have been utterly ridiculous if I had gone back to the breast surgeon to find out I needed to return to the same location for yet another test and another delay in treatment.

Over the next two weeks, there were more diagnostics tests, with the full set of results put in the hands of the doctors for review. After reviewing the results, the chemo doctor confirmed I had Stage 3 Inflammatory Breast Cancer. She stressed the aggressive nature of this cancer type and recommended we proceed with treatment as quickly as possible or risk the chance of it advancing to Stage 4. I knew there might be a chance of cancer progression. From the time my symptoms began in mid-January to this final confirmation of the diagnosis in April, it had been nearly three months.

After confirmation of the cancer type and stage, things started moving more quickly. My chemo doctor requested I schedule surgery to have a port (or port-a-cath)installed as soon as possible so that chemotherapy treatments could be administered.

I met with the breast surgeon and scheduled the next available window for surgery. It was an outpatient surgery that occurred in the morning. They would administer my first chemotherapy infusion the day after this surgery.

My Cancer Team:

- Hematology Oncologist
- Radiology Oncologist
- Breast Surgeon
- Plastic Surgeon

Survivor Secret: What You Need to Know About Diagnostic Tests

- A listing of the doctor appointments that need to be scheduled and the order of scheduling provided by the breast surgeon and nursing assistant

- A list of the diagnostic tests they are going to order and the tests other doctors might order

- The suggested time it should take to schedule the diagnostic appointment and the expected timeframe to receive the results.

They may not have all the answers, but with the answers they do provide, you can create a matrix and timeline for upcoming appointments. They may be able to point you to the other medical professionals who are better suited to answer your remaining questions.

Be friendly with the nurses, technicians and other support staff. In the business world, you gain a lot of information from your informal network. In the same way, you need to develop a similar network for your cancer journey. There is a lot of useful information that can be gained based upon the knowledge of support staff, which can provide an edge in your cancer treatment.

It is not just the cancer patient who is impacted by cancer. Family members and friends are also profoundly affected by this terrible disease. It places a hefty load upon a caregiver. In my case, both my husband and mother alternated roles as primary caregivers.

I was incredibly blessed to lean on and depend upon my husband, Keith. It was easy to recognize I was not the only one hurting because of this diagnosis. It pained me to see my family members in such anguish and feel I caused that distress. What helped me to get through this period was their constant assurance that everything would be okay and their attempts to weave in as many moments of hope as possible.

The role of the caregiver is crucial, and we should not take it lightly. You never know when your world will take a drastic turn and having someone available who will be there for you no matter what is paramount.

Words from a Caregiver: Husband (Keith)

"When my wife was diagnosed with cancer, my initial response was not one of fear or concern. I was not overcome with sorrow or fear; there have been so many technological advancements in cancer treatments. I did not feel the need to be concerned.

However, that mindset changed drastically in just a few brief hours. They diagnosed my wife with Inflammatory Breast Cancer (IBC). Neither of us had ever heard about this type of cancer, so we researched it. IBC is one of the rarest forms of breast cancer, and it is usually not diagnosed until it is in Stage 3. What that means is that it is challenging to treat. Those diagnosed with this form of breast cancer have only a 30% chance of survival five years beyond diagnosis.

At that point, everything changed for me. A flood of different emotions overtook me. A 30% survival rate?! At some point in the next five years, I would watch my wife die, and there is nothing I can do about it. Most importantly, I thought of our children and what her loss would mean to them. How would I be able to keep my emotions in check to ensure that I could be there for them when she passed away?

If you are reading this book, I hope you believe in a higher power because prayer got my family and me through. I eliminated my wife from the picture and placed all the emphasis on me, all the things I promised her and all the things that we could not do as a family. At the lowest moment of my life, I did the only thing that I knew how to do, and that was to pray.

I prayed my wife would be saved, but I also prayed that the Lord's Will be done. At that moment, God spoke to me. He told me my wife would be okay, and he had a plan for her. I got off my knees, went to my wife's side and told her that tonight we cry, tomorrow we attack. Cancer would not defeat you, and God has a plan for this trial in your life.

At that moment, my job was to be a caregiver, mentally and physically. The things we did together, cooking dinner, taking our kids to their practices and activities, etc., would now be my responsibility alone. We got ourselves together and went downstairs to inform our kids of my wife's diagnosis. We explained to them what cancer was, and that it was something that we had to get out of mommy's body. We told them mommy would get worse before she would get better. After some of us cried, we prayed and prepared for the battle ahead.

Being a caregiver is about sacrifice. You are a servant first; you cannot emphasize self, but sometimes, you will need an outlet. Everything is about the patient; how they are doing, is there anything they need, what help can we offer? It is imperative to take offers of support.

As a caregiver, you want to be there to do any and everything your loved one requires. However, if someone is willing to come in, cook, or deliver a meal, stay with your family for a few hours, take advantage of it. You may not want it, but take it; you will need some time to decompress. Being a caregiver is stressful, complicated and time-consuming, but it is worth it. Take your role seriously; you are one of the most critical pieces of this process.

In the days and weeks following my wife's diagnosis, it became clear that her battle would be long and the road ahead, difficult. While traveling this road, I knew she would have some good days and experience her fair share of bad days. In retrospect, deep down, I knew I would have my own battle to contend with. For the sake of our children, I felt I could not allow them to see me having a bad day. I had to show them I believed their mother would be okay. In my mind, the kids needed to see my strength through this adversity, not just for them, but for my wife.

I remember sitting alone in my office and reminiscing about a conversation I had with my father-in-law before my wife and I married. I promised him I would let nothing happen to his little girl. Now, the little girl he raised, the woman that completed me, the woman whom I swore to protect, even with my life, was fighting for hers, and there was nothing I could do about it. I could not protect her from this.

I had to realize there was a real possibility my wife would not survive this ordeal, and in my spirit, the promise I had made my father-in-law would be all for naught. That tore me apart inside more than anything else; I was utterly broken. A child he had raised since birth, entrusted to me to love and protect, could be gone. Had that happened, in my mind, I would have failed him.

After just a few short weeks, I was exhausted physically and mentally. With all the emotions, the stress of taking care of three kids, work, homework, and sporting events, I realized I was not taking care of myself. Men are programmed to be providers; it was my job to provide for my family, financially, physically, and emotionally. I never complained; I just kept those emotions bottled up inside of me, refusing to show weakness. I did not understand the toll it was taking on me mentally.

Even though physically, I was not going through what she was; I was in the storm's midst with her. Looking back, there are two things I would have done differently. One would have been taking part in individual and family counseling. We were extremely fortunate to find an outlet for our children, which allowed them to express how they felt in group therapy.

An outlet was also available for me, but I chose not to take advantage of it. I made excuses because I knew that opening up to someone and releasing those emotions would make me vulnerable, and as a man, I was taught never to show weakness or defeat.

Second, and most importantly, I would have allowed my children to watch their mother battle this disease. Her fight was an inspiration to many people that were suffering and undergoing a similar ordeal. Had we lost her to this dreadful disease, I should have allowed our children to watch her combat it, head-on so she could stay here with our family. Their lasting image of her should have been her fighting. They needed to know their mother did not give up on life or them."

Part 2

I BECOME A
SELF-ADVOCATE

CHAPTER 5:

I Build a Circle of Support

The support my family and I received while undergoing cancer treatment was tremendous. From the outset, we had the support of family, friends, church members, and even youth sports teams.

When I was initially diagnosed, the first people we told were our parents. Those were two tough phone calls involving a lot of tears. They asked what they could do to help and prayed while waiting for confirmation of the treatment plan before determining their next steps.

We were so fortunate to have my parents travel from the Mid-west to be with us. They planned to stay with our family for an extended period. They still worked full-time and had the support of their employers to use the Family and Medical Leave Act (FLMA) provision to take an unpaid leave of absence. Having live-in support from my parents, in-laws, and a special aunt was a tremendous help for our immediate family.

After letting our kids know what was going on with my health, we told friends, co-workers, and church members about my cancer diagnosis. After hearing the news, many of them offered to help in some form or fashion.

The world doesn't stop when undergoing cancer treatment, and it didn't stop for us. Right after my diagnosis, basketball playoffs for the local youth recreation league that our oldest daughter was in were scheduled to start, and my husband was her coach. Her team made it through the playoffs and won the championship game! We had to celebrate, and I offered to host the team celebration at our house.

When I told my friends from church, they couldn't believe it and asked if they could help. They set up everything and cleaned up afterward. I was so thankful for their support of my desire to have some fun times and normalcy while going through this ordeal.

No one should face cancer alone, but at a time when support is needed the most, some people feel the most alone. Feeling vulnerable, they won't ask for help, but being surrounded by a support system can give them the confidence to speak up and let someone else know when something isn't okay.

I considered my care team to include both those who could physically be with me and those who were far away. One of those team members was my younger sister. We are six years apart in age, and growing up, that age difference did not lend itself to us being remarkably close.

Now that we are adults, we are the best of friends. Although we are over a thousand miles apart, anytime we talk, it's as if we live next door to each other. We are not afraid to express our feelings to one another, and I counted this as a significant advantage for me while going through cancer. In her own words below, my sister shares how she felt upon hearing the news of her big sister's cancer diagnosis.

Words from a Caregiver: Sister (Delisa)

"Not so sure of the date, or even the time. A mind-numbing, emotional race to nowhere. An account in my life that I'll never forget. I was selfish.

Sitting in Chick-fil-A and we received the third phone call from my sister. I answered the phone because I am sure she just wanted to check on the unborn baby and me. Ray and I sat at the table as I received the news. "I have been diagnosed with Stage 3 breast cancer."

Overwhelmingly shocked, hurt, numb…. Shocked, hurt, numb. I didn't know what to say, or what not to say; I am pretty sure I said, "when does treatment start and are we seeking a second opinion… WHAT KIND OF CANCER is that, and what does it mean? The next thing I know, I said," Let me call you back."

A flood of tears I didn't want to be heard through the phone. I was sick. Sick of being at Chick-fil-A, sick of living so far away, sick of always having bad things happen to me. I was selfish. Why does God think I need to go through this? What have I done, and what can I do to prove to him I am worth his love and sacrifice? What has my sister done to deserve this?

The whys and the potential outcomes made me mad as hell. I was angry. I was hurt. I was sick!! My thought process moved to now what? How do we go on? Oh, and Google became my new best friend; Breast Cancer No Lump…..Breast Cancer No lump…Inflammatory Breast Cancer. Terrified of the potential outcome because what I was pulling up on the worldwide web wasn't positive.

Later that night, I laid in bed picturing birthdays, holidays, graduations with me standing in her place. How would the kids go on with life without the other half of their pillar of love? All I could think of was death. Why was death the only outcome in my mind?

It wasn't until 3-4 weeks later that I even thought she would make it past the first weeks of chemo. Sixteen miserable weeks of chemo. I hated she would go through that!!!! I doubted God, and it showed; He was testing my faith and unselfishly loving me, her, us through it all.

Our phone calls became more frequent, from 1 to 2 times a week to every day. Most days, it was to say she just had chemo, and she was feeling okay. Or to say she just left the doctor, and the tumor WAS RESPONDING TO THE CHEMO AND THE RADIATION. I doubted God. What an unselfish account of Love he showed to us by giving us His only son. Yet, here I am, doubting God has the healing power of the Almighty.

My thoughts overwhelmed me daily. How was I supposed to be supportive from so far away? I felt useless. I felt as if I was losing my sister. I felt as if this was it. The end was near, and it was too soon. I told no one, not even my husband, I was hurting…. SELFISHLY LOVING HER."

Survivor Secret: How to Create Your Circle of Support

Reach Out to Family First: You may have family living nearby who can assist with household needs and appointments. Family members who are far away can help by talking with you over the phone, sending encouraging notes or helping to coordinate appointments over the phone.

Younger, computer savvy family members can help complete online forms for appointments, or maintain a private family web page or support site so that other family members can stay informed about progress on treatment.

Close Friends Can Help: If you don't have family members or they have limitations in the support they can provide, turn to close friends. Call up a friend and let them know what you are going through. If they offer to help you, take them up on the offer and assign them activities similar to those identified above.

Church Groups: Some religious groups have a Care Ministry or Team that can assist those who are facing an illness.

Support Groups: A favorite resource of mine is support groups. There are website groups and social media sites centered around specific cancer types. Information exchanged on these sites can be valuable. They are filled with people who are facing challenges similar to yours. Some may be further along in their treatment and can provide insight into what they did to overcome a problem they had during treatment. A support group does not have to be limited to in-person meetings. It is because I took part in a social media group that I located the leading doctor for my cancer type and reached out to him to schedule an appointment.

Consider Professional Counseling: Going through such an experience can be very traumatic. You may consider reaching out for professional counseling support. Several associations offer counseling services over the phone and can share details about in-person counseling options based on recommendations from other survivors in your area.

How to find the right support group for you:

1. Start with your local cancer center and ask the cancer navigator or support personnel if there are any local support groups in which you could take part. If there are no groups, see if they will help you start a group.

2. Reach out to local cancer nonprofits. Often, they host support group meetings or may connect you with other survivors in the area.

3. Conduct an online search for organizations that provide support for your specific cancer type. Contact those organizations and inquire into any support groups they host or groups they recommend, either in person or online. They may also have insight into private, closed groups on social media that may be beneficial to you. Should you find any such social media groups, send a message to the administrator and inquire into the makeup of the group, the amount of engagement, and how it's managed.

Cancer Support Resources

- Cancer Support Community: www.cancersupportcommunity.org

- Cancer Hope Network: www.cancerhopenetwork.org

- General Cancer Support Groups: https://www.cancer.net/coping-with-cancer/finding-support-and-information/general-cancer-groups

- Cancer-Specific Resources: https://www.cancer.net/coping-with-cancer/finding-support-and-information/cancer-specific-resources

CHAPTER 6:

Becoming an Empowered Patient

I honestly believe one of the biggest reasons I am alive today is because I was a staunch advocate for MY health. I wanted to understand everything, so I could be knowledgeable about the decisions I would have to make. However, I was extremely surprised by the number of choices I would have to make during my cancer journey.

The entire process was rather frustrating. I was making health decisions, yet I had not attended medical school. How could I know I was making the best decisions for myself? I wondered why I was paying the medical staff for their 'expert' opinions and recommendations if I was making all the decisions? I thought it was ridiculous to have a life and death decision in my hands when less than a month earlier, I had never heard of Inflammatory Breast Cancer.

I took the stance that if they left the decisions up to me, they would have to explain everything in painstaking detail. I'm sure I was one of those quasi-frustrating patients because I asked a lot of questions. But they had the medical training behind them; I did not.

I recall something my dad, an educator, used to continually tell me when I was growing up and attending school as a child. He would say to me that the teachers were there to teach me. If I didn't understand something they were saying, I needed to raise my hand and ask for clarification. If they refused, I was to let him know because it was their job to make sure I understood what they were teaching.

I approached my health with this same attitude. The doctors had to explain it to me or point me to the resources that would help me figure it out. It showed my doctors that I cared about my health and my life, so they needed to provide the same intensity of care. I held them accountable for helping me make informed decisions about my health.

I also knew I didn't have to go it alone. If my husband and family didn't understand something, they would ask questions too. All the doctors got to know me on a personal level. They realized that I counted on them. If I didn't think they were providing me with the information I needed, I would let them know.

Case in point, there was a time when I looked for a second opinion regarding my treatment, which had the support of my current oncology doctor. I sought the advice of the foremost leader in Inflammatory Breast Cancer. I sent him my medical records for review and analysis and followed up with a face-to-face appointment. After his review and physical examination, he recommended a change to my chemotherapy regimen. The regimen would be more aggressive than my existing treatment plan. My primary oncologist was concerned with that approach, asked questions about the second opinion, and wanted an explanation of why it would be the best course of action.

I informed my oncologist that I was not the expert in understanding why the second doctor recommended this change but would appreciate it if the two of them could get on the phone, discuss the recommendations and get back to me with a joint proposal. As suggested, they did just that. When I returned a day later, the second opinion had been accepted, and my local oncologist changed the treatment regimen.

I could have tried to help negotiate my treatment between the two doctors, but I knew I was not equipped with the knowledge or information to broker such a discussion. I set the expectation that as oncology professionals, they should be able to have a worthwhile conversation on my behalf and provide me with the results of the discussion. I did not care if they operated out of two separate oncology practices in two different states. Thankfully, they met my expectations.

I didn't know it, but I was following a recent trend in self-advocacy. Dr. Lynn Eldridge writes in her article, "How to Be Your Own Advocate as a Cancer Patient,"[4] that self-advocacy is like being an empowered patient. Traditional medicine is undergoing a shift to "participatory medicine. "Patients are actively working alongside their physicians to choose the best course of cancer treatment."

During my treatment, I met another cancer survivor and came to admire her efforts in self-advocacy.

She was comfortable in frequently sharing her cancer journey on social media. Her stories offered concrete examples of how one should self-advocate. I was curious to know how she came to be such a strong self-advocate and asked if she would share the importance of patient self-advocacy to readers of my book, and she agreed.

Words from a Self-Advocate (Dara)

"Growing up, my personality was mostly shy, quiet, and introverted. Most of the time, I was uncomfortable asserting myself and dreaded confrontation of any kind. I came out of my shell in college when I realized it was the way to make friends and to be successful in school. Little did I know, this would be the start of my personality shift, becoming someone who would genuinely need to have these skills for what I was to go through with a cancer diagnosis.

---

4   Eldridge, "How to Advocate for Yourself as a Cancer Patient."

I was the first person in my family ever to be diagnosed with cancer. At 39, after being informed I had breast cancer and entering the world of doctors, hospitals, & treatments, it quickly dawned on me that I was the only person who truly knew what I needed throughout the process. I also realized that I was the one who had to use my voice to make sure I received proper care and to ask for the things I needed along the way to help the entire process go as well as possible for me.

This realization helped to transform my personality into being a robust personal advocate for my care. I "self-educated" and researched everything I could about cancer to learn and understand the complexities of this disease. It allowed me to have good medical discussions with my providers because of my knowledge, and it strengthened my resolve always to expect and ask for the care I felt I needed.

I've stayed in hospitals multiple times because of surgeries, and I've had hospital stays because of occasional lousy side effects from treatments. So, I've become very familiar with the ins and outs of medical care, its processes, and the people involved in the medical professions.

I've had wonderful doctors (physical therapists, nurses, medical assistants & orderlies, etc., but I'll just use doctors for the ease of reference) and awful doctors too.

When discussing doctors with others, I sometimes say, "They're simply human too, they just went to school longer than the rest of us," which, honestly, I appreciate and respect the work it takes to become a doctor or other medical professional.

However, as much as they learned in school; sometimes, they must also be willing to learn from their patients. As patients, we get help and information from our doctors. Still, when things go wrong with our medical care, it's critical that as patients, we speak up so that mistakes can be noted, corrected, and even learned from by people in the medical professions.

I always strive to tell the exceptional doctors that they're great and thank them because it lets them know I genuinely appreciate them for who they are and how they treat me.

As for the awful doctors, if it's a minor issue, I will tell them in person. Sometimes, I won't go back to them, or I'll send an email if it warrants their attention. If I find a truly terrible doctor, I'll inform their supervisor. Once, when it was multiple doctors in a top cancer center, I wrote a letter to the President.

I've "fired" a chronic pain doctor for "telling me what I should do" and then walking out without a discussion of what I wanted; a physical therapist for being downright rude and ugly to me when I showed up 5 minutes late and explained it was because of car trouble and this was my first visit to her office. An oncologist who told me I could go back to my first cancer center. My case had been transferred to his cancer center, as being a locally advanced disease was beyond the first institution's realm of care. This happened during treatments for my initial cancer diagnosis.

And I "fired" a whole cancer institution when I was being dismissed as "not having a problem" (it, thankfully, turned out to be a benign mass in my thyroid) by multiple doctors in one well-known cancer hospital.

This is also known as "institutional arrogance." It means the first doctor who didn't want to help me passed the negative vibe on to the other doctors in the same facility when I was trying to get someone to help me with my disturbing & painful symptoms that were being caused by my thyroid.

Even recently, I had elective but necessary surgery for my eyes. My eyelids were impairing my peripheral vision and needed to be corrected by a plastic surgeon. When I went for the surgery, I informed the staff that I have lymphedema in my right arm from having had breast cancer, as I've had multiple areas of cancerous nodes removed. I was even wearing my lymphedema sleeve & hand glove to show they should not use my right arm for any blood pressure checks or needle sticks, as this is proper care for this condition. The staff also put an alert bracelet on this arm for me.

An orderly came in and started to put a blood pressure (BP) cuff on this arm. I said, "No, I have LD." I had the IV in the opposite arm, also not suitable for a BP check, and so I said, "Put it on my calf." She said, "Uh, I have to go check with somebody and left." She returned with the anesthesiologist, and the anesthesiologist proceeded to "lecture me" on "why it had to go on my calf." I said, "I know, that's what I said to her." It irritated me at this happening, but as I was about to be rolled back for surgery, I "let it go" at that moment.

For this surgery, I also asked for a "warmer" blanket on the IV arm before getting the IV. It helps the veins to "show better." I also asked for a lidocaine spray, cream, or shot before the IV to help lessen the pain of the IV being started. These are things I've learned along the way, but they are not the "standard of care. In my opinion, they should be.

Anytime a patient's experience can be made easier, better, and less painful, it should happen automatically and not have to be requested, in my opinion.

So, a week after I'd recovered and feeling better from the eye surgery, I went back for my follow-up visit with the surgeon, but I didn't complain to him about the issue, as he's an excellent doctor! So, of course, I also told him he's incredible and thanked him.

What I did, however, was to stop by the nursing station, and I left a note describing what happened, how I was upset about it, and that all staff needed to be reminded about proper care for patients with different medical needs. I also asked for a supervisor to contact me via phone or email.

To be clear, whenever I'm letting people know something has gone wrong, I'm never screaming or cursing, and I give myself time, first, to "let go" of any anger and frustration at being mistreated. This is so I can be more "matter of fact" in spelling out what went wrong and to inform them about what, if anything, I'd like to have done to remedy the situation.

And, many times, my going back and letting them know they were awful isn't "just for my peace of mind," but because I am very aware that these caregivers are treating many, many patients. And some of these patients, like I "used to be," may be "unwilling, unable, or uncomfortable" to speak up and tell the doctors and staff someone has mistreated them.

To me, patient advocacy means I stand up, not just for "myself," but for everyone else, too, because when you're a patient you don't feel "strong and well," and the people attending to our needs need to be sure they strive to be the best that they can be.

They need to be their best, not just for our sake as patients, but for their own sake too! Because horrible things can and do happen when proper care isn't given, and lawsuits against medical personnel are also a consequence of inadequate health care.

I'd like to remind the unpleasant medical staff people to remember that they wouldn't want to be treated poorly if they were the patient, as compassion and empathy are truly an essential component of the caregiving professions & process.

More importantly, however, I am extending my truly heartfelt gratitude and thanks to those who have provided excellent care for myself & others.

In conclusion, genuinely excellent and wonderful medical care is indeed an essential and integral part of the process in helping patients to recover and be well again.

It is also, in my opinion, highly critical to give compassionate medical care to a patient that is dealing with a terminal diagnosis."

Cancer Self-Advocacy is a critical and essential skill for cancer patients and survivors. Just like many other skills in life, it is one that can be learned. One resource is the Cancer Survival Toolbox,[5] a self-advocacy training program developed in a collaboration between the National Coalition for Cancer Survivorship, the Association of Oncology Social Work, and the Oncology Nursing Society.

According to the National Coalition for Cancer Survivorship, "the program contains a set of basic skills and special topics. True stories of actual cancer patients inspire each scenario. The Cancer Survival Toolbox is for people at any point in their care. It is used by patients, health care professionals, individuals or in support group settings." It is available as a free audio podcast on iTunes.

Another resource is an article titled Survivorship Perspectives and Advocacy.[6] In it, the authors explain that "by implementing survivorship care plans and directing their patients to survivorship resources, health care providers can advocate for survivors and teach them to be effective self-advocates."

You can become a better self-advocate, and it begins with the first step to seek help to become more active in learning how from these valuable resources.

---

5   "Cancer Survival Toolbox."
6   ascopubs.org/doi/10.1200/JCO.2006.06.5300

CHAPTER 7:

My Search for Clinical Trials

After the initial set of consultations with all of the doctors on my cancer team, I followed up with my hematology oncologist. I asked if there were any clinical trials I could consider before treatment began. In my mind, clinical trials would give me access to the latest and greatest medicine to fight this disease. She told me that she had looked at the clinical trials in her clinic, but there were none for which I was qualified.

Hearing her response, I assumed it was about all clinical trials. Now, I realize I had missed an important caveat, which was the part about clinical trials offered through their practice.

As a patient, who was new to this "cancer thing," I assumed she had checked every available source, and there was nothing available for me to consider. It was not until months later that I realized her answer was only regarding clinical trials available through her medical practice and not all trials available throughout the entire U.S.

There are clinical trials available to participate in both during and after treatment. There are even trials available for individuals who have never had cancer. It's often a misnomer that you must have cancer to take part in a clinical trial or that you only use a clinical trial as a last resort. That's not true.

Some clinical trials focus on the prevention of cancer, and some study lifestyle comparisons to determine if certain life choices increase the risk of cancer. I entered a clinical trial following active cancer treatment. They collected DNA samples from me and requested information about my family to determine if there were any perceived linkages in family history, environment, and cancer type. The patterns determined during this trial could help establish predictors of cancer for future cancer patients.

After performing extensive research, I learned that once cancer treatment has begun, it limits the number of clinical trials in which you can take part. That's because many clinical trials want participants to start the trials with a clean slate. Having prior treatments could affect the results of the clinical trials.

Victoria Forster sought to find out "why only 8% of cancer patients in the U.S. participated in clinical trials?"[7]

In the past, it was thought that patient reluctance to participate in clinical trials was a significant factor in the low level of participants. In a joint research study by Columbia University and the American Cancer Society, they found that over half of the patients didn't have a trial available to them at their cancer treatment location. According to the study, about a quarter of the respondents were deemed ineligible to participate in a trial in which they applied. But when offered a chance to participate, half of them did. Ultimately, the study found structural and clinical barriers were the reason that nearly 75% of patients did not participate in trials.

I ran into a similar issue in that I later found a clinical trial I thought I would be eligible to participate in and found out they could not enroll me because I had to attend in-person at the institute. In my opinion, the types of tests they needed to perform could have been completed by my local physician. I can understand their reluctance for remote participants because they perhaps could not ensure the proper controls were in place.

---

7   Forster, "Why Do Only Eight Percent Of Cancer Patients In The U.S. Participate In Clinical Trials?"

Now, I make it a habit to ask about clinical trials at my cancer checkups. During one such visit, I learned about an available clinical research trial. It was a study of cancer survivors, which only required me to have the clinician draw a blood sample, complete some medical history forms and consent to have DNA testing with the results. About nine months later, I received the DNA results via mail.

If they deny you entrance to a clinical trial, find the contact information for the clinical trial and call or email, requesting to speak with someone about the denial of entry. During the discussion, try to get information on the reason for the rejection. With this information, you can then discuss the details of the denial with your oncologist and ask if they can assist with appealing the denial.

The doctor's help could be in the form of a letter to the clinical trial administrator, providing additional test data, or even calling to speak with one of the principal investigators of the clinical trial to see if they can grant a special exception for entry. Sometimes, a one-on-one discussion between medical professionals who understand the clinical trial landscape can help move matters forward quickly.

Survivor Secret: How to Find Clinical Trials

One hurdle to accessing a trial is getting access to information about the trials. The American Cancer Society (ACS) provides an excellent summary of how to find a clinical trial. They explain that there is no one source for all cancer clinical trials, but several resources that are categorized into clinical trial lists and clinical trial matching services.[8]

---

8   "How Do I Find a Clinical Trial That's Right for Me?"

Sources of clinical trial lists include:

- The National Cancer Institute (NCI), which lists government-funded clinical trials

- The National Institute of Health (NIH), which has an even more extensive database with trials that go beyond cancer

- CenterWatchSM, which identifies both industry and government-sponsored trials

- Private companies, including pharmaceutical and biotechnology firms.

Clinical trial matching services are computer-based services used for locating clinical trials. ACS provides some recommended questions you can ask to find a matching service that works best for you. One example of a clinical trial matching service is EmergingMed.com.[9]

Their website states, an individual "can fill out a short questionnaire to identify clinical trials looking for your specific diagnosis, stage and treatment history from the full national database of cancer treatment trials from all sponsors."

A nonprofit organization, SHARE Cancer Support,[10] has teamed up with Emerging Med to offer clinical trial matching services to women of color from underserved communities, such as the Latino, African American, and Caribbean communities.

---

9 app.emergingmed.com/emed/home
10 "Breast & Ovarian Cancer Charity | SHARE Cancer Support."

An abundant source of information regarding clinical trials is available through the National Institute of Health (NIH), which is an agency within the U.S. Department of Health and Human Services (HHS). NIH has an extensive database that houses information on clinical trials available throughout the U.S. This public database is accessible to anyone and can be used to conduct your own search for clinical trials.

Admittedly, when I used the database to search for trials that would be useful for me, I did not find it to be very user-friendly, and the information presented did not appear to be in layman's terms. I felt like I needed to have a medical degree to interpret the information being presented to perform a worthwhile search.

If only there were a service available where you could complete a personal profile, and the system would automatically submit inquiries on your behalf for entry into clinical trials. It would have been beneficial if such a system existed at the time of my diagnosis.

CHAPTER 8:
Cancer Navigators

Cancer Navigators should become part of your village as early as possible in your cancer journey. All creditable cancer centers will have a cancer navigation system in place to assist you during treatment. Cancer Navigators can be one of the best resources to connect cancer patients to local communities and regional and national resources. Most major cancer centers now have a process to initiate a meeting between a patient and a cancer navigator on staff.

Unfortunately, some of us don't know how to use a cancer navigator during our treatment or that they even exist. I didn't engage a cancer navigator until my treatment was almost complete.

I met with a nursing assistant to gather details on scheduling my initial consultations. She shared with me that there were cancer navigators who were available in the local hospital should I need any assistance.

From that brief informal conversation, I did not understand the capability of the cancer navigator as a significant source of support, nor how I was to use them throughout my cancer journey. Instead, I struggled in scheduling my follow-on consults over the next couple of weeks.

Nearly a month into treatment, I had significant engagement with a cancer navigator, who was the facilitator of the cancer support group session I'd attended. A Cancer Patient Navigator[11] is an individual trained to help identify and resolve real and perceived barriers to care, enabling patients to adhere to care recommendations and thus, improve their cancer outcomes.

I liked how she listened, offered words of encouragement, and promised to follow up with participants who needed more help. Her office was near the radiation oncology office, and when I had daily radiation treatments, I would often stop by to chat about what was going on in my world.

Cancer Patient Navigators have proven to be so effective that the "Commission on Cancer (CoC) accredited cancer centers across the U.S. have been asked to meet the American College of Surgeons' CoC Patient Navigation standard. As of 2015, they require this new standard for accredited programs."[12] Because of this standard, every major cancer center has a Cancer Patient Navigation (PN) Program. The range of tasks they provide can vary, but the goal is to ensure that "good health care is accessible, affordable, available, appropriate, and accountable."

According to the Cancer Patient Navigator Tasks across the Cancer Care Continuum, "Cancer patient navigators may be professionals (e.g., nurses and social workers), paraprofessionals (e.g., community health workers), or recognized community leaders and peers (including cancer survivors)."

I recommend you ask your oncologist to connect you with a cancer patient navigator. If such a resource is not available, the American Cancer Society Patient Navigator Program can speak with you one-on-one and connect you with a patient navigator at a cancer treatment center.

---

11 Braun ,"Cancer Patient Navigator Tasks across the Cancer Care Continuum"
12 "Cancer Patient Navigator Tasks across the Cancer Care Continuum."

CHAPTER 9:

Cancer Disparities Can Complicate Treatment

I would be remiss if I did not talk about cancer health disparities. In speaking with one of the expert doctors in my team early on, something he said lingered with me for quite some time. He mentioned that he would take extra care of me because not only was Inflammatory Breast Cancer rare, but when diagnosed at an early age and being of African descent, there were additional risks related to survival. I didn't understand why until later. Understanding these risk factors and known disparities allowed me to make more informed, risk-based decisions with my care.

If you are a person of color, you must be mindful that there are cancer health disparities. You may wonder, what is a Cancer Health Disparity? According to the National Cancer Institute (NCI), "Cancer affects all population groups in the United States, but certain groups may bear a disproportionate burden of cancer compared with other groups."[13]

We can track this disparity based upon several measures, including the number of recent cases, death rate, cancer-related health complications, survivorship following cancer treatment, and many more. After I was diagnosed, I soon learned something very troubling, which was backed by research studies.

---

13 "Cancer Disparities - National Cancer Institute."

CancerQuest[14] summarizes what I found succinctly in that "regarding breast cancer, though white women have a higher incidence of breast cancer, African American women are more likely to die from the disease." According to the National Cancer Institute (NCI), this could be because of "a lack of medical coverage, barriers to early detection and screening, and unequal access to improvements in cancer treatment."

NCI considers several factors to contribute to this disparity and "reflect the interplay of socioeconomic factors, culture, diet, stress, the environment, and biology." For instance, "members of minority racial or ethnic groups in the United States are more likely to be poor and medically under-served (that is, to have little or no access to effective health care) than whites. Limited access to quality health care is a major contributor to disparities."

Why is it vital for you to be knowledgeable that cancer disparities exist? According to CancerQuest, if one can "understand what types of disparities exist and why they exist - patients can find their best fit for treatment." Also, from the American Cancer Society's Annual 2016 Cancer Facts & Figures Report,[15] "social inequalities exist, including communication barriers and provider/patient assumptions, (which) can affect interactions between patients and physicians and contribute to miscommunication and/or delivery of substandard care."

As a patient, I was quick to let a doctor know if I didn't understand what they were communicating. I would ask them to write their instructions or findings. I requested them to direct me to an article I could read, which may better explain what they were trying to articulate. Both you and the medical professional must work together to find an approach for communicating and break down any barriers.

Cultural Competence, as a factor in health disparities, is a topic of national concern within the NIH National Institute on Minority Health

---

14 "Cancer Disparities | CancerQuest."
15 "Cancer Facts & Figures 2016 | American Cancer Society."

and Health Disparities (NIMHD). The NIMHD is responsible for the establishment of standards in healthcare, related to cultural competence, and in 2013 released an update to the National Standards for Culturally and Linguistically Appropriate Services (CLAS) in Health and Health Care.[16]

These standards and guidelines are in place to ensure "the provision of health services that are respectful of and responsive to the health beliefs, practices, and needs of diverse patients can help close the gap in health outcomes." I highly recommend you become familiar with these standards, one of which requires healthcare professionals to provide language translation services.

Through grants awarded by the NIMHD, organizations are receiving federal government funds to research cultural competence in healthcare, such as the National Center for Cultural Competence (NCCC) at Georgetown University.[17]

NCCC explains, "the compelling need for cultural and linguistic competence," with one of those reasons being "to improve the quality of services and health outcome." In their study of Cultural Competence, they state, "despite similarities, fundamental differences among people arise from nationality, ethnicity, and culture, and from family background and individual experience." These differences affect the health beliefs and behaviors of both patients and providers.

Some states, like the state of Maryland, are enacting legislation to address this challenge, and some non-profit organizations, such as the Visiting Nurse Service of New York, have tailored programs to provide culturally appropriate care to help eliminate health disparities. In the state of New York, they were the first home healthcare organization to launch multi-cultural programs to serve their diverse communities better.

---

16 "What Is CLAS? - Think Cultural Health."
17 "NCCC | Home."

Survivor Secret: Keep Medical Notes

As a cancer patient, you must understand your diagnosis and treatment protocol before leaving the facilities. At a minimum, ask for a copy of the medical notes that are a summary of the appointment, and if there are any specific diagnoses or instructions provided during the doctor's visit, ask for those instructions to be printed out and given to you before departure. One excellent practice is to keep personal records and information that could be reviewed with a family member and relayed in subsequent appointments with other medical practitioners who may need an account of your visit.

Part 3

HOW TO HANDLE SHOCK, ANGER, AND FEAR

CHAPTER 10:

Turning "Woe is Me" into "I Got This!"

When faced with a devastating cancer diagnosis, you experience a variety of emotions. You have a choice in that you can let these emotions get the better of you or you can seek ways to let these emotions energize you into taking action in fighting this disease. Who better to share her fighting spirit than a U.S. Air Force Veteran and 2-time cancer survivor, Tanja Thompson, and how she overcame a series of major life obstacles.

Words from a Survivor: Retired Air Force Senior Master Sergeant (Tanja)

"My life as a 2x breast cancer survivor will never be the same as it doesn't dominate my existence, but beneath the surface, it's there peeking in plain sight with the scars across my entire torso, the fading shadow port scar above my chest, the uneven breast and without a nipple or areola. Breast cancer was just one of the stops of my life's journey. I know all too well of hurt, pain, and the unbearable trials and tribulations that keep me grounded. Because of my strong faith in God, I am better, stronger and wiser and have gained enormous strength in finding and being comfortable with SELF.

I can remember the day like it was yesterday, it was a sunny May day in 2005, a day no different than any other morning other than stopping by Andrews Air Force Base(AFB) to get my mammogram results before heading to work. While getting dressed in my military blue service uniform, I remember my husband asking, "Tanja, do you want me to go to your doctor's appointment?" I looked over my shoulder and said, "No, sweetie, after the appointment, I'm going to head into work." Driving to the hospital on Andrews AFB, I was thinking about the wonderful spring break vacation with the kids driving down the California East Coast Highway.

When I received the first breast cancer diagnosis, I was 42 years young, active-duty, and didn't know anyone personally with breast cancer. The only person remotely familiar was a military colleague whose sister had died from the disease. I was shocked and floored when I heard the words, "Mrs. Thompson, you have breast cancer." Sitting in her office all alone, my body went limp, my mind was numb, not hearing or processing those death words. She said you have ductal carcinoma in-situ (DCIS) in the right breast and infiltration of the cancer cells in the left; the cancer was in multiple quadrants of both breasts. The recommendation was a bi-lateral mastectomy with skin-sparing, immediate placement of expanders for reconstruction, but no chemotherapy, radiation, or tamoxifen. By the end of May, my breast was gone, and so was cancer. The likelihood of a recurrence was extremely low, at least that's what I was told, less than 3%. While attending a breast cancer support group at the Pentagon, someone said, you are so lucky that you don't have to worry about a reoccurrence. That statement was true for five years when it was no longer the truth. In 2010, I discovered a lump in my left breast, and this time, the cancer was invasive.

From a military patient perspective, the support that was made available to me was slightly different from the first and second diagnoses, largely due to diagnosis, type, treatment and my outlook on the disease. The reason I say this is because in 2005, my breast cancer diagnosis and treatment was a bi-lateral mastectomy with no radiation or chemotherapy, and it actually took me a long time to accept I even had breast cancer – I was in denial, secrecy was paramount, I never cried, and I didn't see myself as a breast cancer survivor, which meant

I didn't need or want anyone's help. I also remember telling my co-workers, colleagues, and staff that my diagnosis was my business and not theirs to tell. I didn't want anyone to know I had breast cancer; I didn't want to be seen as that airman (an enlisted member in the Air Force) with breast cancer.

In 2010, I had the full gamut: multiple surgeries, Trams Flap reconstruction for the left breast, chemotherapy, radiation, and several different hormone treatment therapy regimens. I can remember saying to myself; I'm going to have fun with breast cancer this time, which meant not being afraid or hiding in a shell. For example, my first chemotherapy treatment was October 1, 2010, and by Halloween, I was completely bald. In celebration of my outlook on life, chemotherapy, a bald head, my family came through for Halloween, and I had my husband put a red arrow down the middle of my head, and I dressed up as Aang, The Last Airbender. To commemorate the loss of my hair, we had a funeral for my hair with a tombstone.

This process has been a journey, and I have learned many things along the way. One of the most important is that breast cancer is no longer a death sentence but an opportunity to live life. I am a true testament that you can survive breast cancer, not once but twice, knowing early detection is the key to saving lives. Below are a few of my "Pearls of Wisdom" I would recommend for living:

1. *Lift your voice. Ensure your voice is being heard; for example, I was unable to take the tamoxifen as the side effects were horrifying. The doctors tried several different types, all with varying side effects. I finally just said, no more, my quality of life was being diminished with all the side effects. I made an informed and conscious decision to stop taking the medication. I do advise before starting or taking any medication to consult your healthcare professional.*

2. *Write down your thoughts. As an introvert, my energy comes from being alone, and I've learned to journal as a young girl.*

My earliest journal, which I still have, is from 1980. During those times of regaining my inner strength, I journaled my entire breast cancer experience, both in written and picture form, which brought me to writing the book, "What to Expect When You Weren't Expecting Breast Cancer." My book shares that life doesn't stop just because you've been diagnosed with this disease, and these scars (internal and external) are a symbol of strength, power, hope, life and an inspiration for others that we are SURVIVORs.

3. *Join a support group. This was the best decision forced upon me by an intervention between my boss and husband. They saw where I was spiraling down a dark hole of depression, anxiety, anger and hostility. The support group allowed me to share with other breast cancer survivors how I felt without having to explain myself. During our sessions, I learned, "I am Enough."*

4. *This is a question and a statement. What's a 4-letter word that haunts us?! It is the word HELP. With that being said, I wouldn't ask and/or accept HELP. For so many of us, especially those that have served in the military, you learn to take charge of a situation. Breast cancer was my situation, and I didn't need anyone's help; in my opinion, asking for help was a sign of weakness.*

I believe we all have a purpose in this life, and everything happens for a reason because God doesn't make any mistakes. During this journey, moving from the darkness into the light, my faith in God grew that much stronger. If you want to get out of the darkness of your tragedy and see the triumph in your life, you have got to plug into different energy. Whatever inner God, whatever higher calling, whatever higher self that is, the way without it is living in the absence of light."

Survivor Secret: Resources for Veterans

- Department of Veteran Affairs (va.gov)

- Homeless Veterans (va.gov/homeless/employment_programs.asp)

- VA Vocational Rehabilitation and Employment (va.gov/homeless/employment_programs.asp)

- VA Care Givers Program (va.gov/homeless/employment_programs.asp)

- Humana TRICARE Military (tricare.mil)

- CaringBridge (caringbridge.org)

- Breast Cancer Awareness (google.com/search?client=safari&rls=en&q=Miltary+and+Breast+Cancer&ie=UTF-8&oe=UTF-8)

- Therm Approach (thermapproach.com/faq)

- Military Benefits (militarybenefits.info)

- 3 Heroes who took the fight to Breast Cancer (militarytimes.com/native/drs-hjf/2019/10/13/3-heroes-who-took-the-fight-to-breast-cancer/)

- Veteran Health Administration (va.gov/health/)

When I was initially diagnosed with cancer, I was in complete shock that I could have the disease. After the shock came fear - fear that I wouldn't be here for my family and live to see my kids grow to become adults. How could this be possible – heck, my youngest son was only three years old! Life isn't supposed to happen like this. Why did my kids have to bear such pain?

Then came another feeling - anger, because I felt like everything was moving too slowly from diagnosis to treatment. I kept hearing the word "aggressive" in my head along with the fact that this form of breast cancer started as Stage 3 with no gradual progression, skipping Stages 1 and 2 and just BAM, I had Stage 3 cancer.

If it was so aggressive and already at Stage 3, why were they taking their sweet little time on starting treatment? On top of that, I felt like my doctors weren't even advocating for me to get my appointments scheduled as soon as possible. Why in the world would you tell someone who has just been diagnosed with an "aggressive" form of cancer that they needed to "wait" for a series of appointments?

I was selfish enough to believe that appointments with people who had less aggressive forms of cancer needed to be bumped. All I thought was if it turns out I had progressed to Stage 4 cancer because of having to wait for these appointments, I would go off, and there would be hell to pay!

Those are just a sampling of the thousands of thoughts swirling around in my head. "Experts estimate the mind thinks between 60,000 and 80,000 thoughts a day. That's an average of 2500 to 3300 thoughts per hour."[18] Eighty percent of those thoughts are negative, and 95% are repetitive thoughts, the National Science Foundation Reports.[19] Negative thoughts were indeed swirling around in my head, and I had to figure out a way to get my mind right.

---

18 Sasson, "How Many Thoughts Does Your Mind Think in One Hour?"
19 Verma, "Destroy Negativity From Your Mind With This Simple Exercise."

It was a stressful time for the two to three weeks between my initial diagnosis and my port installation. I had a sense of dread about starting chemotherapy, and then came a sense of relief when the chemotherapy treatment began. This was because there would no longer be any more delays because of medical appointments.

Next came the fear and doubts the treatment would work and that I might die. What would happen to my family and my kids? How would they be able to survive without me?

I Join Local Support Groups

Thankfully, I concluded I could not hold on to all those feelings and stay sane. I located and joined a local breast cancer support group. The support group was free to join with no cost to the patients.

The group met weekly in a reception area of the local hospital radiology center. It was not a large room, so it felt cozy and more personable. Just before the start of the meeting, they placed chairs in a circle, so everyone could face each other. We sat in the circle and discussed topics facilitated by a Cancer Nurse Navigator employed by the local hospital system.

This Navigator served in one of two such positions at the hospital to field questions throughout the day from patients, hold one-on-one counseling sessions with patients or family members, and facilitate weekly support group sessions in the evenings.

There was one support group for newly-diagnosed breast cancer patients or who were undergoing treatment for the first time. A second session on an alternate date was for women facing late-stage cancer or a recurrence. It was very thoughtful to separate these two demographics because each had unique challenges and associated questions.

During a meeting to share my concerns with one of our children's school dean, I learned she was a breast cancer survivor. She shared that there was another parent in our school community that had survived IBC. She offered to connect us, and I said, "yes." It turned out that we lived less than five minutes from each other.

It was through this new connection that I learned of another local group whose members also had this "rare, aggressive cancer." The group met regularly at local restaurants, and I joined them. My circle was further expanded to include hundreds of more women in a private community group on a popular social media platform.

There, I learned how to find the best doctors, what symptoms I could expect to have, and how to cope with the struggles of fighting against this disease. Because I reached out for help, I learned about stylish lymphedema sleeves from Lymphdiva ®, an expert doctor in Philadelphia to possibly add to my cancer team and advice on whether I should entrust my care with a surgeon that had done very few operations with an IBC patient. By the way, the answer was no!

I asked, how would I go about choosing a surgeon with significant experience operating on IBC patients? The suggestion was that I ask the expert doctor in Philadelphia. I emailed his office, and the nurse practitioner got back to me with the name of a local oncologist in the DC area, who also specialized in IBC.

I contacted her office with this weird request. I asked if they could recommend the surgeon she used for most of her breast cancer patients, especially those who had performed surgery on patients who had IBC. The receptionist took down my question and got back to me the same day with a recommendation for a new surgeon.

I met the new surgeon about a week later, and we immediately clicked. I look back on this culmination of events and honestly believe that if I hadn't taken the first step to speak with the dean at my kids' schools, I might not have reached where I am today.

This example shows the power of networking and how the benefits extend well beyond the business community. Finding someone who has been through similar challenges with the same cancer has significant advantages. The experience they have and the wisdom you can get is invaluable.

I Encounter Caring Nurses

Aside from the support groups, I often came into contact with several nurses who would do their best to lift my spirits. Many nurses helped me to maintain my sanity.

There was the nurse who comforted me when I thought I wasn't getting adequate testing done and prayed with me after a test procedure. There was a nurse who listened to me plead to have the doctor provide me with a recommendation for another doctor to perform surgery, even though I was not their oncology patient.

My Church Community Steps Up

I had many thoughts about death. While I did not fear death, I feared the aftermath for my family and how they would handle things if I were no longer here. One Sunday, after attending church services, I began crying after having thoughts about deserting my family. My pastor came over to comfort me and led me to a group of Elders for prayer.

After they prayed over me, one of the women Elders talked with me and uncovered my fear of not knowing who would take care of my family if I were gone. She shared how less than ten years ago, she had been diagnosed with a brain aneurysm and only given a 10% chance of survival.

I thought, wow, that was a smaller chance of survival than what I was facing, and she's alive and well here, right now, speaking in front of me. She told me she had similar fears about her sons back then and what would become of them if she were to pass away. She said through prayer, she could release those feelings and be comforted that her Lord would be there for them.

I Discover Online Support Groups

For additional support, I turned to social media and joined a support group for women with the same rare breast cancer as I was facing. This online community opened my eyes to the struggles and successes being met by other women. It inspired me when I came across good news stories, but I would get to feeling down when I came across some incredibly sad stories.

Those sad stories affected me so much that my mom took notice and inquired about what was making me feel so distressed. I told her about the social media site, and she encouraged me to turn it off because I needed to protect myself from negative thoughts while trying to heal. I followed my mother's guidance (she also is a licensed counselor), and I felt much better.

My experience with online and in-person support groups was equally rewarding, and they both had their benefits. The benefit of the in-person support group was the ability to hear directly from others about what they were experiencing and ways they were overcoming obstacles like mine. They also provided suggestions for local resources that may be useful for others in the same geography.

Because I had a rare form of breast cancer, the online support group was a phenomenal addition to support my mental health. It was a social media group that had restricted access and administered by individuals diagnosed with the same cancer. The suggestions were more specific, and women were able to respond at all hours of the day and night. I connected with many of the women online.

Sometimes, women could arrange in-person meet-ups to communicate at a local level. The local meet-ups were great. I had an opportunity not only to meet ladies that were still going through treatment, but I also met women in remission from IBC. This gave me hope.

Something that inspired me to think more positively was diving into a book written by Lynn Eib titled, "50 Days of Hope." I can remember it like yesterday. I downloaded the book onto my Kindle device and started reading it while we were on a family road trip to the beach. I was both happy and sad. It delighted me that we were going on a road trip with my family, many of whom had flown from another state to join in the fun together. I was also sad because this was a change to the original plan.

Before my diagnosis, we'd planned to meet and enjoy a week in Myrtle Beach, SC, for a family vacation. However, because of my regimen for chemotherapy treatment, I could only be away for a maximum of 3 days. Because of the risk of infection, I could not swim in the ocean or even the swimming pool. We decided to go to Virginia Beach, which was only 3.5 hours away from home.

I was feeling down on myself because I was the reason the family had to take a detour on our family vacation plan. Here I was, heading on a road trip to a beach, and I wouldn't even be able to get in the ocean with my kids – I could only watch them from a distance.

I buried my sour face in the book on the ride down to Virginia Beach. Oh, my goodness! The stories were so inspiring and genuinely gave me hope that everything would be okay. I think reading that book had the single most significant impact in turning around my perspective from "Woe is me" to "I got this!" There were more bumps along the way, but I celebrated the good times and did my best to dwell less upon the bad.

Sometimes, people will try to keep their cancer diagnosis to themselves. You don't have to share specific details of your treatment with everyone, but sharing this information with others and letting people know you are seeking individuals who have had a similar experience can be the information sharing that leads to improved treatment outcomes.

I Start a Journal

My brother reached out to me and asked what I needed. I told him I had read somewhere that it was good to use a journal at this time. A few weeks later, a box showed up in the mail from my brother's fiancé, and inside, I found a pink leather-bound journal and a book related to fighting cancer.

In the past, I hadn't been the type who would write in a journal every day, but I committed to giving journaling a try. I would write in the journal during various windows of time. It did help to write some of my feelings down. Sometimes, I would write and cry. Other times, I would write about successes or having reached a milestone during treatment. I'm still writing in my journal all these years later.

"Research shows that writing 20 minutes a day for three months will produce long-lasting benefits to your physical and emotional health. Journaling can help you sleep better, reduce fatigue, and help you adjust psychologically to a cancer diagnosis and treatment."[20]

I wish I had been able to stick to a routine and journal every day. No matter what, I just couldn't find my rhythm. I later learned about a technique called Guided Journaling, which "is a self-reflective process, allowing participants to access deeper levels of self-knowledge, based on a set of prepared questions. The reflection is spontaneous and hap-pens just by writing down the thoughts that emerge at the moment

---

20 Fellow, "Journaling Your Way through Cancer | MD Anderson Cancer Center."

(instead of first thinking and reflecting, and then writing down the reflections)."[21]

Christine Bergsma is the creator of a guided journaling system called Journaling Through Life (www.journalingthroughlife.com). She has a series of journals, Journaling Through Breast Cancer (specific for breast cancer survivors) and Journaling Through as Support (designed for friends and family of those with cancer).[22] These journals provide anyone dealing with this life-changing event the opportunity to gain insight for themselves to be of genuine support to the person with cancer and those around them.

This and other guided journals for cancer survivors, such as "Cancer ... and I: A 365 Day Guided Diary to Journal Your Cancer Emotions" offer a way that therapist and author Ronell Grobler says "will quickly become a repository for the things you can't say to anyone else —even yourself."[23]

---

21 ch, "Guided Journaling — Collaboratio Helvetica."
22 "Journaling Through Breast Cancer: Bergsma, Christine: 9780986965531: Amazon.Com: Books."
23 "Cancer ... and I: A 365 Day Guided Diary to Journal Your Cancer Emotions: Grobler, Ronell: 9781518619199: Amazon.Com: Books."

CHAPTER 11:

Finding Support for Caregivers

I was not only concerned about my mental health but also about the mental health of my family members. My husband was very supportive of me and took excellent care of our family and me, but I worried about how he was feeling and his spirits as I received treatment. He did not have to go through the physical therapies, but I knew that seeing me go through this was taking a toll on his spirit.

I encouraged him to go to a support group for caregivers, but he didn't want to do so. Instead, he poured himself into making sure that not only was I okay, but our kids were doing well too. Looking back, I wish there had been a way to convince him to take part in a caregiver's support group. I just couldn't find the right words to make it happen. A helpful book I recommend for caregivers is titled, "Things I Wish I'd Known: Cancer Caregivers Speak Out" by Deborah Cornwall.

She includes a section on caregiver healing and believes "that these kinds of action programs allow them to overcome negative feelings about what the cancer experience may have taken from them and to focus on dealing with their feelings about that experience in a constructive and even nourishing manner."[24]

I regret not taking advantage of one-on-one counseling for myself and each member of my family. I don't know why I thought group

---

24 Known, "Cancer Caregivers - Things I Wish I'd Known - Resources."

sessions, reading inspirational stories, and my religious practices would be enough.

If each of us had our own counselor, it could have helped us come to terms with what was happening more quickly and enabled us to more effectively transition into our new normal after completing active treatment in November 2013. There have been several struggles during and after that period for which counseling could have provided the tools for us to navigate more effectively.

Survivor Secret: Where to Find a Support Group

Several organizations can help you find a good cancer support group. The Cancer Hope Network[25] has a service to match you with someone who can speak with you over the phone when you need cancer support.

The American Society for Clinical Oncology[26] outlines the benefits of joining a support group to include the various types of groups. There, you can find a group right for you.

Thinking back to my diagnosis and having the surgeon sit down with me to discuss the cancer team, I believe I would have scheduled an appointment with a counselor or psychologist if she had shared how they would be an integral part of my team.

25 "One-on-One Support for Adults Impacted by Cancer."
26 "Support Groups | Cancer.Net."

Below is a list of resources to support mental health, both during and after cancer treatment:

- Cancer Support Communities provide free individual support to cancer survivors. (cancersupportcommunity.org/)

- Sharsheret is an organization that offers psychosocial support over the phone to women who have had breast or ovarian cancer. (sharsheret.org/)

- An article with useful tips if you are striving to have a positive attitude with cancer: verywellhealth.com/how-to-keep-a-positive-attitude-with-cancer-2248819

CHAPTER 12:

Pay Attention to Your Children's Mental Health

Our kids were ages 11, 7, and 3. The oldest was in her first year of middle school as a 6th grader; our middle child was in the 3rd grade, and our youngest was in pre-kindergarten. After receiving the diagnosis, the scariest thing I faced was telling our children I had cancer.

With the "take charge" attitude that already existed within me, my husband and I decided to quickly tell our kids what was going on with their mom, even though we didn't have all the answers. We knew that it would be discussed often in the next few weeks, and we didn't want to risk them finding out from someone other than the two of us.

We called a family meeting the day after I was diagnosed to communicate to our kids the best way that we knew how that "Mommy has cancer." That it was a disease that the doctors would treat, and they would see a lot of family and friends over the next few months to help Mommy and Daddy. There may be times that Mommy wouldn't feel well enough to do the usual things that they would expect me to do. There were not a lot of questions during that discussion; just a lot of hugs and saying, "I love you."

With concern for the mental health of our children, we signed up the two oldest for group sessions for kids at the local cancer support center. The group was comprised of children whose parents were actively in cancer treatment. Unfortunately, our pre-kindergartner was too young for the program. The sessions were held once a week for six weeks. During the sessions, the kids worked on an arts and crafts project while the two counselors explained cancer at the level a child could understand. The sessions were far from home, but we had family members to help with transportation and the offer of support from close friends.

At one point, our kids had a project where they were using a coloring book that had flowers and weeds in it. My youngest daughter told us that Mommy's cancer was like a weed next to a pretty flower, and the doctors were trying to get rid of the weed but still let the beautiful flowers grow. I was glad she shared this with me because it showed she'd absorbed what the counselors taught.

During the next few years, our middle child underwent an extreme growth spurt. People commented on her height, insisting she 'was growing like a weed.' This would upset her, and she would kindly tell people she wasn't growing like a weed but was growing like a pretty flower. That response let me know the group sessions had a lasting positive effect on her understanding of cancer.

You quickly learn that life goes on while fighting cancer. As a young adult cancer patient starting treatment during the second half of my children's school year, we were uniquely challenged with ensuring our children had the mental capacity to handle this life-changing event along with the activities of a regular school kid.

We had to make sure their respective schools knew what was occurring in our home and ensure they had the right amount of support. We knew it might affect their grades and social activities because of what they might be feeling and wanted any changes to be monitored by the school personnel and communicated to us quickly.

The school personnel we met with were supportive, but looking back at that period, I realize we only communicated to the school leadership. It would have probably been even more useful to meet with their school guidance counselor, social worker, and any other school-based mental health professionals and specifically ask for recommendations to ease our children's burdens during this time.

I thought it was imperative to reach out and make sure everyone was on the same level regarding our children. We did the same thing at our childcare centers. In regular times, it's challenging to juggle family schedules, and that gets magnified when a parent is undergoing treatment.

The owner of the childcare center our two oldest attended after school recognized this and offered to help by taking them to dinner and their group therapy session on a day that conflicted with one of my chemotherapy treatments. The group sessions were almost 20 miles away, much farther than the regular daycare pick up at our local schools. In these instances, we brought our village along for the ride, and they stepped up like none other.

Survivor Secret: Mental Health Resources for Children of Survivors

- How to Talk to Your Preschooler About Cancer. cancer.net/blog/2018-04/how-talk-your-preschooler-about-cancer

- Talking with Teens About Cancer: cancer.net/coping-with-cancer/talking-with-family-and-friends/talking-about-cancer/talking-with-teens-about-cancer

- Talking with Children About Cancer: cancer.net/coping-with-cancer/talking-with-family-and-friends/talking-about-cancer/talking-with-children-about-cancer

Even if your children are adults, it will still be challenging to tell them you have cancer because you may not want your grown children to have any mental anguish in contemplating the future because of your diagnosis.

Paula K. Waller said as much in her article titled, "Communicating Cancer to Adult Children"[27] and provides several recommendations on this challenging step. Two interesting recommendations were to be honest and to let them help. This help can come in the form of both physical and mental help. One suggestion that hit home, regardless of the age of your children, was to "use your diagnosis as a way to teach your children how to navigate a medical crisis – how to be a self-advocate.

---

27 "Communicating Cancer to Adult Children | Patient Power."

Part 4

MANAGING EXPENSES

CHAPTER 13:

Disability Insurance

A little over a year before my cancer diagnosis, a thought from a conversation that happened ten years prior came to mind. If anything were to happen to me, did I have adequate insurance coverage? It was 2012; I had just started my company in October 2011. I strongly felt that I needed to start coverage for both long-term and short-term disability and life insurance.

I distinctly remember a conversation my husband and I had back in 2001 with our financial advisor. The advisor quoted a fact about disability close to the statement below:

A 35-year-old has a 50 percent chance of becoming disabled for 90 days or longer before age 65. About 30 percent of Americans ages 35-65 will suffer a disability lasting at least 90 days during their working careers. About one in seven people ages 35-65 can expect to become disabled for five years or longer.[28]

When I heard this staggering statistic, it stuck with me. I only had two people in the company at that time and didn't know if my company could qualify for this insurance.

I reached out to my financial advisor and expressed this concern. He indicated that with a company my size, I could set up an individual

---

28 "CDC: 1 in 4 US Adults Live with a Disability | CDC Online Newsroom | CDC."

life insurance policy and long-term disability, but we could not establish a short-term disability plan.

Because I had such a small company, the insurance companies would require an extensive check into my medical history, a physical exam, and blood work. It was a lengthy activity that got frustrating at times, but I was finally approved a few months later. The combined monthly insurance rate was not as low as the one I'd paid when working for a large employer, but it gave me peace of mind that it was in place.

After my diagnosis was confirmed, and the extensive cancer treatments began, the side effects left me unable to work at 100%. Because of the aggressiveness of the cancer, it was designated as one that required compassionate care. As a result, I automatically qualified for Social Security Disability Insurance (SSDI).

Some people think that since they have private short-term or long-term disability coverage, they don't qualify for social security benefits. Anyone who has paid into the social security program is eligible to apply to the program if you cannot work due to an illness.

Applying for social security is a very cumbersome experience. You can either go to a social security office to apply for social security disability insurance (SSDI) or complete an online application. If you do not feel comfortable completing the disability application alone, consider asking a family member to assist you. If you are computer savvy, I suggest you complete the online form as it may take some time to get an in-person appointment through your local social security office.

In both cases, filing for long-term disability through my insurance and the Social Security Administration required the completion of an extensive amount of documentation. The information necessary included all medical doctors and hospital visits from the onset of the disability to the present day, including their contact information, dates of prior appointments, and authorizing the release of my medical records. A list of prescription medications was also required.

It was a lot of data collection, and although cumbersome, having the information organized was beneficial. The disability insurance company sent out a representative to interview in-person to gather details on the limitations I had with working full-time while undergoing treatment. From this interview, the representative would then file a report, and I had to wait for an official determination whether I qualified for payment of disability insurance benefits.

I realized later that there were a lot of things in my disability insurance policies I never paid attention to until I needed it. I learned about waiting periods – the number of days from diagnosis to the point one qualifies to receive disability payments. Depending on the policy, that waiting period could start from the date of diagnosis, while others start on the date of submission for the claim. Some waiting periods are 90 days, and others can be six months. For this reason, I recommend you submit a claim as soon as possible.

Another interesting fact I learned, which was a significant relief, was that once they declared me disabled, the private insurance companies waived payments of premiums.

Thankfully, both insurance claims were accepted upon the first and only submission, with no rejections or appeals required. Some processing took longer than others. And, sometimes, one approval hinged upon the approval from another plan. For example, because they approved me for Social Security Disability Insurance, it was difficult for private insurance companies to deny my claim.

The Social Security Administration has field representatives who can assist with completing the SSDI application. For private disability insurance applications, consider reaching out to a trusted organization, such as the Patient Advocate Foundation, who has representatives that can provide case management help, which includes helping to identify a resource to assist with completing the private disability benefits application.

Understand that once a submission is made, it may take weeks to receive an approval or denial letter and the associated amount to be paid. Last, if you have children, then you may also qualify for additional SSDI benefits to cover childcare expenses while disabled. This application will be initiated after you have received your approval of SSDI benefits. Note: although it may take some additional processing time, they base the eligibility upon your approval date.

Sometimes, a disability claim is denied. All insurance companies have an appeals process. Look carefully to see if there are any restrictions on the appeals process. For instance, should you appeal and are denied, be sure this one appeal was not your only option.

In either case, you may obtain professional help from a lawyer who specializes in disability claims or a company specializing in this area, such as a Disability Advocate. A Disability Advocate is a non-attorney with legal expertise but without a law degree.

Once I completed treatment with the SSDI, I was eligible to return to work gradually, which allowed me to keep SSDI payments for that return to work period. For private disability insurance, the payments stopped as soon as I returned to work on a part-time basis.

Survivor Secret: Disability Insurance Resources

- Social Security Disability Insurance (SSDI)

- Online Application - ssa.gov/onlineservices/

- Compassionate Care Allowance (Automatic Approval) - ssa.gov/compassionateallowances/

- Disability Insurance Learn Center - policygenius.com/disability-insurance/disability-insurance-definitions/

- Patient Advocate Foundation - patientadvocate.org/explore-our-resources/preserving-income-federal-benefits/about-disability/

CHAPTER 14:

Prescription Drugs

Before treatment, I underwent a series of diagnostic tests and attended multiple medical appointments. The medical bills had not started arriving yet, but we knew they were coming. With the completion of diagnostic testing, my oncologist was finally ready to deliver the treatment plan to my husband and me.

The treatment plan called for two series of chemotherapy treatments. The first set would be administered weekly, followed by a second set, which would be administered bi-weekly but in more substantial dosages. The first series of chemo treatments would be followed up the day afterward with a shot that would reduce the risk of infection and the likelihood of having to be admitted into the intensive care unit (ICU). The shot increased the white blood cell count, which tended to become dangerously low following a chemotherapy infusion. These shots allowed me to maintain acceptable white cell blood count levels and continue subsequent chemotherapy treatments.

With this treatment plan in place, one of the office managers asked to meet with us to review the full cost for the chemotherapy treatments. My husband and I sat across from the office manager, and she broke down the costs for the chemo treatments and office visits.

I would need Neulasta booster shots. These shots would boost my white blood cell count, so I could avoid a trip to the intensive care unit (ICU) and have to receive a blood transfusion. They would ensure my white blood cell counts would remain high enough to withstand the next infusion.

What came as a sticker shock was the price of the shot. It was over $5,000 per shot, and there would be six of them. The look my husband and I passed to each other was one of disbelief because we knew we had no choice but to pay the price.

That's when the office manager told us about a program offered by the pharmaceutical company. If we filled out some paperwork, they would waive the costs between the co-pay ($25) and the insurance deductible until we reached our out-of-pocket maximum. Once that threshold was reached, the insurance company would cover 100% of the costs. We had an absolute look of relief and thankfulness after hearing this news. We did not think we qualified for any prescription drug benefit program because we had a moderate income and health insurance.

Survivor Secret: Always Ask About Prescription Drug Programs

Many people may think prescription drug programs are only offered to individuals unable to afford the cost of the drugs. Those programs exist, and some programs are not limited by family income.

The office manager found the program she offered to us with a search engine, such as Google Search. She put the name of the prescription drug into the search field, and a few keywords, such as drug benefit program for "insert drug name," and the search engine returned a few possible benefit programs. She then researched those programs and found the benefit plan suitable for patients in their oncology practice. We were so thankful for her due diligence in finding this program.

Using search engines can be a useful way to find prescription drug benefit programs for cancer patients. Since learning of this practice from my oncology practice business manager, we have used this same technique to find drug benefits for other prescriptions used by family members. We have been successful in finding some enormous benefits for dermatology prescriptions, which are often not covered by our insurance plan.

Below, you'll find a sample list of Prescription Drug Assistance Programs as found on the Susan G. Komen website.[29]

- CancerCare – Co-payment Assistance Foundation (cancercarecopay.org)

- CancerCare – Komen Treatment Assistance Fund (cancercare.org/financial/information)

- Medicare (medicare.gov/)

- NeedyMeds.com (needymeds.org/pap)

- Patient Advocate Foundation (patientadvocate.org/)

- Patient Advocate Foundation – Co-Pay Relief Program (copays.org)

- Partnership for Prescription Assistance (pparx.org/)

- Rx Hope (rxhope.com/)

- Strings for a Cure (stringsforacure.org/SFAC-Programs/)

---

29 "Breast Cancer Prescription Drug Assistance | Susan G. Komen®."

Pharmaceutical Relief Program

The Pharmaceutical Research and Manufacturers of America (PhRMA) provides a search engine of financial assistance resources for patients. Their tool can be found here: medicineassistancetool.org/

CHAPTER 15:
Travel During Diagnosis and Treatment

Local Travel for Treatment

Many patients are required to visit multiple doctors on multiple occasions to seek cancer treatment. Those in rural areas have an even more significant challenge. There is a shortage of family doctors in those areas, which means there is a shortage of specialists like oncologists. As a result, to seek cancer treatment, many patients must go a significant distance to get cancer care. Longer distances can delay diagnosis or influence the choice of treatment. In this chapter, I will not only share my routine for accessing cancer services, but I will also share how I overcame the challenge of seeking cancer treatment far away from home.

Fortunately, living in a major metropolitan area, there is a multitude of medical providers in the immediate area, and my oncologist, radiologist and surgeon were not very far away.

When coordinating my treatment plan, I understood that I would require support with transportation for some appointments, especially following chemotherapy treatment and surgery. Thankfully, the only part of my treatment that would require overnight hospital stays would be the surgeries.

For my weekly chemotherapy infusion session, a family member or friend would accompany me to my appointments. The infusion sessions were typically 4-6 hours in duration. Sometimes, I would have one person drop me off, and another come to pick me up to take me home.

Depending on the chemo infusion, I would sometimes have to get checkups both before and after the infusion. The checkup before infusion was a blood draw to confirm that my white blood cell count was high enough for me to proceed with infusion the next day. The visit to the office the day after the infusion was required when I had to have the Neulasta chemo booster shot.

Radiation therapy treatment sessions were daily, Monday through Friday, for 33 total treatments. Each appointment would last about 30 to 45 minutes, with much of that period waiting to be called back to be radiated. I was fortunate enough to drive myself to these appointments because the only immediate side effect following radiation was fatigue.

If I needed transportation to make it to these local appointments, I could rely upon my husband, friends, or family members who were in town to support our family. I have since learned that in emergencies, the American Cancer Society has a ride program called Road to Recovery,[30]

which "provides transportation to and from treatment for people with cancer who do not have a ride or cannot drive themselves."

Long-Distance Travel for Diagnosis

Since the beginning of my cancer diagnosis, I wanted to ensure that I had access to the best doctors to treat my form of cancer. Due to it being so rare, I assumed there might be some unique challenges and nuances with the treatment approach.

---

30 "Road To Recovery."

In the online support groups, I discovered that there were very few experts for this type of cancer. At the time a preeminent expert for my cancer diagnosis was at a University-based hospital in Philadelphia, Pennsylvania. Because I was nearby in the state of Virginia, I decided to visit and seek a second opinion from this doctor.

Because this visit was occurring over the summer, we had the flexibility of bringing our children with us. We loaded up the minivan and took the 3-hour family road trip to Philadelphia. We made a conscious decision to make this a mini-vacation for our kids. While I went in for my appointment, our kids hung out with their Dad sightseeing in downtown Philly. When I finished my appointment, I rejoined my family to continue the weekend. For this quick trip, we only had to cover one overnight hotel stay, gas, and food expenses.

I took a couple more trips alone to visit with the expert in Philadelphia and then in Chicago when that doctor changed hospitals.

The chemotherapy regimen he recommended was different and more experimental than the one prescribed by my local oncologist. Although it would have been covered by insurance in Philadelphia, it was not necessarily covered by insurance at the private practice back home.

For me to take advantage of his recommendation, it looked like I would have to make weekly trips to Philadelphia for infusion. Traveling such a great distance every week would have been very taxing on me physically and my family emotionally and financially.

Recognizing this was something I wanted, my local oncologist went to bat for me with the insurance company and got approval to modify the treatment regimen and have it administered at my local oncology office. It was a blessing to have the two unaffiliated doctors work together to satisfy my desires for treatment and eliminate the need for travel. It was the best scenario for my family and me.

Long Distance Travel for Surgery

Three years after starting treatment, I reached the end of a long journey and embarked on the last portion of my treatment plan, plastic surgery. Because of the type of cancer treatment I received, this surgery would also require an extremely high level of expertise that narrowed my search for available doctors.

I finally found a plastic surgeon who specialized in this procedure. However, working with him would require me to travel to New Orleans, LA. The length of stay and the distance required a lot more planning. We would have to stay there for over a week. During a planning call with the New Orleans medical facility, the associate asked if we would like to have some guidance on how to prepare for our stay.

She asked if we had booked a hotel. I told her we had not and if she had any suggestions to send them our way. She indicated that a local branch of the American Cancer Society had a facility in the metro area, called the Hope Lodge. It was not too far away from their downtown surgery center and was free to cancer patients regardless of their stage of treatment. They had limited availability, and they reserved it on a first-come, first-served basis.

She offered to assist us with the application to book the facility if we were interested. I immediately responded with a resounding yes, and she sent me a partially completed form, asked me to complete the remaining fields, and submit it to the local American Cancer Society office for processing.

It was not guaranteed we could stay at the facility because of the number of requests, but at least we had the option available to us. Less than a week before departure, they approved us for our stay at the Hope Lodge. The only transportation cost we had to cover was the flight, which we paid for with airline miles, and the rental vehicle.

We searched for options to cover our airfare, but our family income exceeded the threshold to qualify for free/reduced airfare in support of cancer treatment. If we could not secure a stay at the Hope Lodge, the surgery center had a list of preferred hotels that offered a slight discount for a visit.

Personal Travel

Sometimes, when you're undergoing cancer treatment, you need a break - time to get away from it all. It can be rather tricky with limited time between treatments or restrictions on the types of activities in which you can engage.

During this period, I had two opportunities to travel for pleasure. The first trip was to a family vacation, which had been planned before my diagnosis. We proceeded with the trip but had to make some adjustments. I was actively undergoing chemotherapy, and we did not want to change the chemo schedule, which could affect my outcomes.

Chemo was being delivered in cycles, and I had maybe six days between treatments. Because of chemo, my immune system was compromised, and I could not go into a swimming pool or the ocean because of the bacteria and risk of infection. My doctor did not want me to be in large crowds and wanted me to be especially wary of being around sick people and small children.

We loaded up a 15-passenger van and took a quick road trip. I was happy we were going but sad I could not get into the water. Instead, I sat with family members on the beach, inside a protective tent, watching my kids have an enjoyable time. I couldn't help but feel good inside to be with my entire family. My flexibility was vital, along with my family's willingness to be flexible.

The second trip I took was with my husband to celebrate our 15th wedding anniversary. Once again, we had to change the original plan.

We'd originally planned to return to Europe for our 15th Anniversary. The last time we had traveled there together was in the spring of 2001, before the birth of our first child.

The restrictions on the length of time we could be away from the cancer treatment limited the distance we could travel. We decided we still wanted to celebrate this momentous occasion, so we decided to go somewhere neither of us had visited before in the states, and that was San Diego, CA.

We checked with my oncologist and knew I would complete my very last chemotherapy regimen just before going on our trip. The only problem was the blood draw that had to occur a specific number of days following each chemo treatment to ensure my immune system was not compromised.

Since we wanted to leave immediately following my last chemo treatment (double celebration for completing chemo and our anniversary), I asked my oncologist if it would be okay to have another company complete the blood draw in the San Diego area. She gave the okay, and I found a reputable company to complete the blood draw while there.

I scheduled the blood draw to take place a few days after our arrival. We hired a taxicab to take us to the location (this was before Uber and LYFT), checked in, completed the blood draw and the paperwork, indicating that the results needed to be sent to my oncologist in Virginia. After that, we took the cab to the San Diego Zoo to continue our adventures.

We rented a car, drove up the coastline, and visited one of the beaches. The ocean looked inviting, but the waters of the Pacific Ocean are frigid. I didn't feel any sadness about not getting into the water.

It took a little more planning, but getting away to have some fun is essential. It may just be for a moment, but it's an excellent opportunity to get your mind off your current situation and enjoy living.

Survivor Secret: Travel Resources

- Cancer Patient Travel: (usairambulance.net/)

- Transportation Resources for Cancer Treatment: (cancercare.org/publications/303-transportation_ resources)

- American Cancer Society – Road to Recovery Program: (cancer.org/treatment/support-programs-and-services/ road-to-recovery.html)

- Livestrong Medical Care Transportation: livestrong. org/we-can-help/planning-medical-care/transportation- and-other-cancer-support-services

- AngelWheels: (angelwheels.org/)

- Lodging & Transportation Resources for Cancer Survi- vors: (pearlpoint.org/lodging-transportation-resources- cancer-survivors/)

- Joe's House (joeshouse.org/), is a nonprofit organiza- tion that helps cancer patients and their families find a place to stay when traveling away from home for medi- cal treatment.

CHAPTER 16:

Mortgage and Rent

One of the most substantial cost-of-living expenses is housing, whether you rent or own a home. If you were already straining to cover your living expenses, getting diagnosed with cancer can make a challenging situation even worse.

As a business owner, my salary was severely impacted because I could not work for an extended period because of treatment. As a result, our household income took a significant hit.

My first concern was trying to make sure I could bring in enough funds to ease the burden on my family and ensure I could at least cover the mortgage. Having this taken care of would help to reduce a significant portion of our financial concerns.

Thankfully, I had the disability insurance plan in place. After filing the disability claim for both my private disability insurance and social security disability insurance, I had enough funding to cover this considerable expense. It left me wondering what my choices would have been if I hadn't had disability insurance coverage.

Mortgage Payments

In an article titled, "Cancer costs: How to manage housing expenses during treatment"[31] by Melissa Brock on Bankrate.com, she suggests homeowners contact their mortgage company to speak with a specialist. Some options to consider include short-term repayments, forbearance agreements, loan modifications, and more.

Additional options to consider include looking for a less expensive homeowner's insurance policy and refinancing or reassessing the value of your home for tax purposes. Before you consider any of those options, check to see if you have mortgage protection insurance for your home, which is not to be confused with private mortgage insurance.

Amy Loftsgordon explains in What's the Difference Between PMI and Mortgage Protection Insurance?[32] the key difference between the two. "They design PMI to protect the lender, not the homeowner. Mortgage protection insurance will cover your mortgage payments if you lose your job or become disabled, or it will pay off the mortgage when you die."

According to Ellen Chang in "Mortgage protection insurance: When you might need it," some policies function as a life or disability insurance. "Policies that pay a benefit for a job loss or a disability typically cover your mortgage payments for up to a year or two."[33]

Some mortgages that are backed by government-sponsored enterprises, such as Freddie Mac or Fannie Mae, can receive mortgage assistance. The U.S. Treasury Dept. offers mortgage assistance through a program called The Hardest Hit Fund, which is available in 18 States and the District of Columbia. For instance, in Florida, they primarily

---

31 "A to Z List of Cancer Support Resources | Cancer Support Community."
32 Attorney, "What's the Difference Between PMI and Mortgage Protection Insurance? | Nolo."
33 Chang, "Mortgage Protection Insurance: When You Might Need It | Bankrate."

offer this funding to assist unemployed or underemployed borrowers with their first mortgage until they can resume full payments on their own, or they pay a onetime fee for a homeowner who has returned to work or recovered from underemployment.

If none of these options work for you, consider reducing the financial burden by renting out space in your home or selling the property to downsize into a less expensive residence. Discuss options to prevent foreclosure with a realtor and/or mortgage representative.

Rental Assistance

Several nonprofits offer rental assistance for cancer patients who cannot cover their existing rental expenses and those seeking short-term housing to get care closer to a cancer treatment center.

The National Cancer Institute provides a listing of over 100 organizations providing support by cancer type. Organizations like the Cancer Financial Assistance Coalition[34] will not respond to individual requests for financial help. When searching the website, enter your zip code, and the site will return several organizations that can assist with housing needs in your area.

To get help, it will typically require you to complete an application. Sometimes, that application will have to be submitted to a social worker affiliated with your cancer center to verify you are actively being treated for cancer.

Another consideration is to reach out to your local government human services department. They typically have social workers who also have a network of contacts, both local and regional, and information on national organizations and programs that can provide rental assistance services.

---

34 "Free Resource for People with Cancer."

Survivor Secret: Programs for Mortgage Assistance

- Angel Foundation

- CancerCare

- Cancer Family Relief Fund

- Cancer Finances

- Cancer Financial Assistance Coalition (CFAC)

- Colorado Housing Assistance Corporation

- GreenPath Financial Wellness

- HealthWell Foundation

- Housing Solutions for the Southwest

- Leukemia and Lymphoma Society

- Neighborhood Assistance Corporation of America

- Operation Hope

- Patient Advocate Foundation

- Triage Cancer

- Unison Housing Partners

- Upper Arkansas Area Council of Governments

Survivor Secret: Navigating Government Assistance Programs

We were fortunate enough to be financially sound and have adequate insurance in place when I was diagnosed with cancer. But it's easy for me to imagine what our circumstances would have been like if this were not the case.

I grew up in Oklahoma, and although my grandparents worked for a living, sometimes, there was not enough money to sustain their families. At one time or another, they had to rely upon government social assistance. Making ends meet continues to be a reality for many people today.

According to a 2017 report by CareerBuilder,[35] an employment website, 78% of American workers say they're living paycheck to paycheck. If you break it down by gender, 81% of women and 75% of men are living this way.

What happens if they diagnose you with cancer, and you are already struggling financially? Some may elect to forgo cancer treatment. Others may find themselves having to turn to government social services and nonprofits during cancer treatment. Does this mean you are destined for a death sentence? The answer is NO! Every one of us as Americans has a right to life and access to life saving healthcare.

Before initiating treatment, a good doctor will have their patients meet with a medical benefits advisor or social worker to provide an estimate of costs for care and assess your ability to pay for medical expenses.

---

35 "Living Paycheck to Paycheck Is a Way of Life for Majority of U.S. Workers, According to New CareerBuilder Survey - Aug 24, 2017."

If the costs exceed what is affordable for a patient, they may offer to provide a discount on their services. If they cannot offer a discount on their services, they may help to identify discounts on the medication through a drug discount program provided by pharmaceutical companies.

Afterward, they may have you meet with the local hospital to determine if they have a cancer navigator who may investigate additional ways to offset the costs. The cancer navigator will review their portfolio of services but may also encourage you to visit your local government assistance office.

Every state has a department that focuses on human services, including healthcare, food, and housing. The U.S. Federal Government provides government benefits, and they describe a summary of those benefits on their Government Benefits website at https://www.benefits.gov/.

Their website has a useful Benefit Finder tool accessible from their homepage. If you have difficulty navigating these services, consider contacting your state or local human services office. Start with their help desk to ask critical questions that were not answered via the Benefits Finder tool. Then determine if you need further help to complete any applications and if so, ask if someone can assist you in completing the forms.

I have heard that some Medicaid patients find it difficult to find providers who will accept their government insurance for cancer services. Through the Health Resources and Services Administration (HRSA), the U.S. Department of Health and Human Services administers programming for Federally Qualified Health Centers (FQHCs). FQHCs are "community-based health care providers that receive funds from the HRSA Health

Center Program to provide primary care services in under-served areas."[36]

They offer free or reduced services, based upon a sliding scale. Some comprehensive services they provide include preventive health services, dental services, mental health, and substance abuse services, transportation services necessary for adequate patient care, and finally, hospital and specialty care.

Some cancer treatment options would fall into the hospital and specialty care services. At our local federally funded health center, they have made arrangements with a local research hospital to provide cancer surgery pro-bono for patients that are referred to them from the local health center. Through this same program, patients also have access to a discount drug pricing program.

---

36 "Federally Qualified Health Centers | Official Web Site of the U.S. Health Resources & Services Administration."

CHAPTER 17:

Childcare Expenses

One unique challenge for people diagnosed with cancer who have young children can be finding reliable childcare services. Before the diagnosis, they may have provided care as a stay-at-home parent. After the diagnosis, that parent may no longer be able to care for their children while undergoing treatment. The additional expense of childcare on top of the rapidly increasing medical costs can seem daunting.

Those who are fortunate enough to live near family members may be able to rely upon them for childcare. Unfortunately, most Americans live over two hours away from close family. In our case, we lived in the Mid-Atlantic region of the U.S. while our family members lived in the South and Midwest parts of the U.S.

What alternatives do you have with limited income and family members who live very far away? There are nonprofit organizations that can cover all or some childcare expenses for those undergoing active cancer treatment. Using a search engine to locate nonprofits, you should be able to find organizations willing to cover childcare costs. If your child was already attending a childcare center, you can ask the provider if they would consider waiving some or all the childcare costs for a designated time.

If you are a member of a religious group or congregation, consider asking them if they may cover some of the childcare costs.

You can also reach out to middle school and high school students looking for volunteer hours who may want to serve as Mother's Helpers. If you are home alone with your children, they could help to serve lunch or watch them play outside during the summer. Relief from some of these students could be useful for short-term support throughout the day.

If you have an extra room in your home, you may consider hiring a nanny to come live with you. There are reputable services that provide them; all that's left for you to do is interview and determine if one would be a suitable fit for your home. We had a neighbor who found a nanny on Craigslist who could provide childcare. You can reduce the expense for a nanny even further if you supply room and board.

Undergoing cancer treatment during the summer with school-age children can be daunting for some children. Without a regular school day to break the monotony, it may be useful to enroll the children in a summer camp.

If these options are cost-prohibitive, seek organizations that can cover the costs or provide services for free. In our case, our church waived the charges for a couple of weeks of summer camp for two of our children.

There is an organization that provides free camps to children of cancer patients and survivors, called Camp Kesum. They host these camps throughout the United States, and many of the camp counselors are former campers who attended the same camp.

There are so many unique situations that drive the need for childcare. A fellow survivor, Austyn Hutton, shares her story, which she hopes can inspire others to be open to sharing their story and asking for help.

"*My name is Austyn Hutton. I'm a stay at home mom of four kids aged 7, 5, and 3-year-old twins. They diagnosed me with cancer in 2016. I was 27 years old and pregnant with our twins. My older two boys were 4 and 2. I found the lump myself when I was 30 or 32 weeks pregnant. It took about a month of doctor appointments before I was diagnosed with Stage 2 breast cancer, ten days before my twins were born.*

Seven weeks after our babies were born, I started chemo. I had chemo for six months. I then had a lumpectomy. They also removed my primary auxiliary lymph nodes to test to see if they had tumors in them. I ended up having tumors in all 6 of the lymph nodes they removed. This bumped me up to Stage 3 breast cancer, with the potential of being Stage 4.

I went back and had 15 more lymph nodes removed from that area. Luckily, only one of those had a tumor in them. I also had my ovaries removed for several reasons. One of them being I would then be post-menopausal, allowing me to take the hormone therapy that my oncologist believed to be best for me. I also had a PET scan with clear results, meaning the cancer had not metastasized.

About a month after surgeries, I started radiation. I had radiation Monday through Friday for seven weeks. After that, I was finally done with treatment. I finished treatment in January 2017, almost a full year after I was diagnosed.

During this time, we still had to take care of our four small children who were then aged 4, 2, and newborn twins. I probably had close to 100 doctor appointments between diagnosis and treatment. It was rough!

Just after I was diagnosed, another one of our friends announced he had a reoccurrence of throat cancer. He and his wife also had young children. In their announcement, he said that if anyone wanted to help, they could contact their "care coordinator" and gave his email address. We reached out to our friends, told them about our cancer, and asked more about what their care coordinator was and how they were helping them. Their care coordinator was a close friend, who acted as a secretary of needs for them.

Anytime someone said, "let us know if you need anything," the care coordinator would get their name and number. People would email and tell them things they were available to do, like bring a meal or babysit their kids. Any needs they had, such as childcare, meals, errands, etc., would be communicated to their care coordinator, who would connect them with the people who had volunteered to help.

We adopted this immediately. We asked around until we found a dear friend who could do this. The key was finding someone available to do this and being honest about what it would include. We asked one friend first, and she wasn't able to pull it off, and that was okay! She ended up helping in lots of other ways.

With our Care Coordinator, Jolee, we created a unique email address that people could use to volunteer to help us. When we announced that we had cancer on Facebook and also to our church, we told people about Jolee and our unique email address. We had many people email to help! Also, any time people said to me, "let me know how I can help," I would send Jolee their information.

We needed A LOT of help. As chemo went on, I needed more and more help taking care of the kids. About halfway through treatment, I needed someone extra at our house every day, helping take care of the kids while I rested, and my husband worked.

It was humbling to accept help from others regularly, but we did it because we REALLY needed it. My body couldn't have healed as it needed to if we didn't have help. We also needed a lot of childcare for all the appointments I had.

I think one reason we had so many people volunteer to help is that we were open and honest about what we were going through. We communicated the needs we had on Facebook, and people volunteered. It helped to use such a public forum like Facebook to communicate updates and our needs.

When I was first diagnosed, a social worker from our cancer center would come and talk to us and ask us about our needs. We were honest with her about what we might need. Our greatest need was always childcare. It turns out they were able to work out a solution to some of our childcare problems too. This has been incredibly helpful AFTER treatment when I have a follow-up appointment. We couldn't use it during treatment because our twins were too young, and our appointments were too long."

Austyn's story is one of perseverance, enduring a diagnosis of cancer while pregnant and then having to undergo treatment while caring for newborn twins. She could have fallen into a depth of despair, but she and her husband did not give up. Instead, they accepted they needed help and sought supporters to assist them during their time of need.

Another thing you should recognize from this story is, even if someone is not comfortable fulfilling a need you have identified, it doesn't mean they could not fill another yet to be identified need.

Survivor Secret: Find Help with Childcare

Having a list of volunteers who can be contacted to support a need is invaluable. One resource to consider is the Nanny Angel Network (nannyangelnetwork.com/), which provides free professional relief to mothers with cancer. They "care for children 16 and under, and offer compassionate support to families throughout treatment, recovery, palliative care and bereavement."

Even if such an organization is not available in your area, check out their service offerings, and consider connecting with local nonprofits to determine if they could provide a similar service in your area.

CHAPTER 18:

Medical Garments and Equipment

One of the most significant unknowns besides whether you will be healed by cancer treatment is the cost for medical care, including medical garments and equipment. During the surgery, I would have a significant number of lymph nodes removed and, as a result, might be at risk for lymphedema. This condition causes swelling of the lymph node system. Because of lymph node removal under my armpit, there could be considerable swelling of my entire arm.

To reduce the risk of swelling, the doctor recommended lymphedema therapy and a lymphedema sleeve. Before surgery, the circumference of my arm was measured, and a specific amount of pressure was determined to be needed by the sleeve to prevent swelling. With this information, I could order a lymphedema sleeve.

This type of sleeve looks like what you see the football or basketball players wear on their arms during games. The sleeve I ordered from a standard medical catalog looked medical grade and medically necessary. In other words, it looked awful! I knew I had to find something that looked more appealing.

I found a company called Lymphdivas®, founded by a woman who had also fought breast cancer and, like me, thought the garment selection of sleeves at the time were undesirable. She discovered that she could use various patterns, combined with the compression technology and have hundreds of design options to choose from. The options are visible on their website, easy to order, and shipped directly to your home.

Survivor Secret: Resources for Medical Garments

Ask for recommendations for medical garments or devices from your local oncology provider, cancer patient navigator, or support group members. If you don't get recommendations from these resources, search online and review the product recommendations. Recommendations proved invaluable for me to find functional and comfortable medical garments for use while undergoing treatment.

- A Little Easier Recovery: (alittleeasierrecovery.org/ index.php?link=features&gclid=EAIaIQobChMIr5 fGv4eT6AIV2MDICh0Quw0AEAAYASAAEgLjrfD_ BwE)

- Choose Hope: (choosehope.com/category/cancer-apparel/)

- Woman's Personal Health: (womanspersonalhealth.com/)

- Care Aline: (carealine.com/)

Part 5

MANAGING MY TREATMENT

CHAPTER 19:

My First Chemo Day

I was way over-prepared the first time I went in for a chemotherapy session. I read something somewhere that I needed to be prepared with reading materials and snacks because it would be a long day.

I went into the session, excited that I would finally start fighting this thing. It was January when I first noticed the symptoms, and now here it was the middle of March, and I was finally being treated.

I kept thinking, if this was so aggressive, why did it take so long for us to get to this point of treatment? Then I remembered it had just been about two weeks since my initial diagnosis. The day before my first treatment, I had outpatient surgery to install a large port under my right clavicle. Now, this newly installed port would be used to dispense my first chemo dosage. It surprised me that I could have a chemotherapy infusion so soon after surgery, but it also relieved me that it could begin so quickly. I was ready!

After checking into the office, they led me back to the infusion room, where there were about a dozen recliner chairs surrounding a glass-enclosed workstation that housed the infusion nursing staff. The chemo room was bright and airy and only had two other patients. Several of the chairs faced large windows that covered three-quarters of the wall. There were also three private rooms for administering chemo.

For the first chemo session, I wanted to use a private room, but they directed me to a place in the open area. The oncology nurse assigned to me wanted me to be in the open area so she would have a line-of-sight view and could monitor my status consistently. She could make sure I was not having any adverse reactions to the chemotherapy dosage.

I brought a plethora of comfort items: a pillow inside a pillowcase specially made by my mom, a blanket, a Kindle device for reading, snacks, and headphones. My husband was also there to keep me upbeat, but I think we were both still in shock that we were in this space, and I was being treated for cancer.

As I prepared for my first session, I had been studying up on what to do to have a smooth day of treatment. I read about the possible side effects I could have, such as nausea or loss of appetite. I also learned about the need to maintain a nutritious diet and drink plenty of fluids. I thought about eating a lot of foods that had health benefits, such as those containing high dosages of antioxidants. But I checked with my doctor, and she insisted I not take any supplements nor focus on a diet high in antioxidants as it might diminish the impact of the chemotherapy regimen. I had to be sure not only to eat healthily but also to avoid foods that could negatively affect the chemo treatments.

The nurses suggested I avoid eating my favorite foods before and during infusion. Chemo can change your taste buds, and eating these foods could cause you to no longer want them. Instead, I thought I would try a new food I had not eaten before. I was focused on being as healthy as possible, so I brought salad, tortilla chips, and hummus.

I had never eaten hummus before, but I love chickpeas on salads. It turns out that eating hummus for the very first time and being administered chemo was not a good idea. When they delivered the chemo, the very first thing I noticed was the smell of the antiseptic, which did not sit well with me and made me nauseous.

Next, they had to clear the port, which entailed taking a saline solution and inserting it into a tube connected to my port. I could taste the saline solution in my mouth even though it was being injected into the port below my clavicle. Adding the chemo dose made my mouth taste like metal.

I got hungry a little later and had some chips and hummus, and it tasted like dirt. To this day, I avoid hummus like the plague because the smell of it brings back memories of that first chemo dosage. Other than the memory of the hummus leaving the nasty taste in my mouth, I remember little from that day. I felt weak and tired, but I think it was more emotionally draining than anything.

Besides eating healthy, I drank plenty of fluids. A few things I learned about treatment: drink fluids out of a glass container rather than plastic or metal; use plastic utensils when eating. I had to test this out for myself. Sure enough, the water tasted different, and using utensils that were metal-based left a metallic taste in my mouth. I followed these recommendations because it was essential to make sure I continued to eat no matter how bad I felt. I needed to make sure I was giving my body fuel to fight the disease and stay as healthy as possible.

So began my routine for chemotherapy treatment; chemo administered Monday or Tuesday, Neulasta shot the next day. Depending on the scheduling, I was pretty much out of commission until Thursday. The Neulasta shots made me feel like I had the flu, accompanied by body aches that caused me to writhe in pain for most of the day. It took about a day to recover from these side effects. I lived for the weekends when there would be some normalcy in my life.

Not long after starting treatment, I started losing my hair. It was something I prayed would not happen, but I undoubtedly knew it would happen. As the hair fell out, it started pulling at my scalp. It became slightly uncomfortable and, at times, unbearable. A few days after my second chemo session, instead of waiting for all of it to fall out, I decided to let it all go.

That evening, I told my husband it was time to cut and shave off my hair, and I wanted the entire family to be involved. My Mom, Dad, and our girls each took turns cutting off strands of braided hair until they were all gone. My husband took a pair of hair clippers, and while the rest of the family watched, he finished shaving my head until it was bald.

Throughout the process, we took pictures, and afterward, I received a hug from everyone. My Dad complimented me on having a pretty bald head, and my son looked up at me and raised his little 3-year-old hands, placed them over my bald head, and told me we now looked the same. This brought tears to my eyes, but I didn't let them drop as I wanted to be strong for my little boy. Having my family there made it seem beautiful. I felt brave and encouraged I could make it through this ordeal.

Survivor Secret: Chemotherapy Considerations

Just like our family, many other cancer patients have gatherings with family and/or friends to contend with hair loss from treatment. They commonly refer to them as Hair Shaving Parties. In her article titled, "Staying Positive and Making Chemotherapy Hair Loss Look Good,"[37] Christine Benney suggested that one could not only host a haircut party but also donate your hair.

---

37 "Staying Positive and Making Chemotherapy Hair Loss Look Good."

"Remember that without your hair to hide behind, your facial features will be allowed to truly shine." Consider accessorizing with scarves, hats, earrings, or a wig.

Going through chemotherapy can be physically or mentally harsh. Receiving gifts from friends and family members to support me during those treatments lifted my spirits. One such gift was in the form of a cancer care basket, created by a local cancer support nonprofit. Ben Ratkey provides the Top 5 Cancer Gift Ideas for Chemo Patients to include a Friend and Family Gift Basket, Gift Sets, and Cancer Head coverings. Examples of gift baskets include a Cozy Blanket and one with essential soothing aides.[38]

---

38 "Our Top 5 Cancer Gift Ideas for Chemo Patients | Choose Hope."

CHAPTER 20:

Surgery

I knew the importance of having a surgeon who had performed the specific type of surgery required by individuals with IBC, at least 100 if not 1000 times. Since my doctor in Philadelphia was an expert in IBC, I reached out to his office and asked for recommendations on a surgeon.

Their initial response was to provide a doctor in the Philadelphia area. With requirements for an overnight stay, expected returns for checkups, and childcare requirements, I asked about a referral in the region where I lived.

They did not have a specific referral but knew of an oncologist at an area hospital in DC. My expert doctor had referred other IBC patients in the past, who'd been unable to travel to visit him for a consultation. They provided the doctor's number and recommended I contact their office directly to get a referral for surgery and to specify they had sent me.

I immediately placed a call to that doctor's office and explained my situation. The next day, I received a call from a nursing assistant in the DC office, who provided me with the name of a local surgeon the doctor recommended. That doctor was at a hospital in Washington, DC. When it came time for my surgery, we could leave our house that morning and drive straight to the DC hospital for surgery.

My parents were able to care for our children while my husband supported me in the hospital, and friends could come to the house and give them relief, so they could drive to DC to check in on me and return to my house the same evening. I stayed overnight at the hospital and returned home the next day. I would undergo routine checkups over the next six weeks. My husband or mom drove me to my appointments and back home the same day.

CHAPTER 21:

Exercise During Treatment

From the beginning, I was glad to have an oncologist who believed in the benefits of physical exercise. When my hematology-oncology doctor asked me if I exercised, my response was I occasionally exercised. She said that was good and suggested I continue to exercise if I could do so during chemotherapy treatment.

She would do her best to kill the cancer, but it would be up to me to maintain my physical health to stay healthy enough to sustain the therapies that would harm not only the bad cancer cells but also some good cells.

The chemo would take a toll on my heart, so it was important to strengthen that muscle. Thankfully, the doctor ordered some tests before chemotherapy to establish a baseline of health for my cardiovascular system.

Studies show that exercising while undergoing cancer treatment can ease the side effects of chemotherapy. In Australia, exercise is recommended as a part of cancer treatment for all cancer patients. It can "counteract the adverse effects of cancer and its treatment." Exercise is promoted by all members of the multidisciplinary cancer team, to include a referral to exercise physiologist or physical therapists with cancer experience.[39]

---

39 Monique, "Exercise as Part of Cancer Treatment - Harvard Health Blog - Harvard Health Publishing."

The National Comprehensive Cancer Network (NCCN) shows that exercise reduces fatigue, with patients seeing a 40% or more decrease in fatigue with regular exercise. If a patient regularly exercises, beginning at the point of diagnosis, it can lower risks of complications during cancer treatment.

It's essential to get approval for exercise from your doctor and even ask for a referral to a physical therapist. Having a discussion with a physical therapist who specializes in cancer before beginning any physical activity will ensure you can get an individualized exercise plan.

My path to exercise while undergoing cancer treatment began with walking around my neighborhood. I wasn't exactly sure how I would feel following treatment, but I started by slowly walking on the day of my chemo treatment. Because I'd received a Neulasta shot the day after chemo, I felt too ill to walk on those days, so I would pick up walking two days after the Neulasta shot.

I also took part in an instructor-led exercise class as much as possible. My local cancer center offered wellness classes, such as yoga, Tai Chi, and moderate aerobics. They geared these classes towards cancer patients and their families. Best of all, they were free. There was also an option for an oncology massage at a reduced cost, where the therapist was trained to work with cancer patients to ease some of the side effects. Treatment may have made exercise tough, but that oncology massage was on point.

Later, when I began the second chemo regimen, I no longer had to take the Neulasta shots. The debilitating feeling that persisted after the shots was replaced by numbness in my extremities. Walking became more difficult, so I took advantage of the Tai Chi and yoga classes.

Dr. Lee W. Jones, in an Expert Q&A about Exercise During Cancer Treatment, explains that "research shows that not only is exercise during distinct types of cancer treatment safe—it can also have several benefits. From decreasing your risk of treatment side effects to potentially making your treatment more effective at destroying tumor cells, moving your body is important to your health."[40]

In fact, "LIVESTRONG at the YMCA, a small-group program developed and established in partnership with the LIVESTRONG Foundation, assists those who are living with, through or beyond cancer to strengthen their spirit, mind, and body.

Recent research from the Yale Cancer Center and Dana-Farber/Harvard Cancer Institute confirmed that LIVESTRONG at the YMCA participants experienced improved fitness and quality of life as well as significant decreases in cancer-related fatigue."[41]

Many cancer centers in the U.S. offer exercise programs geared to cancer survivors. Some organizations provide fitness programs designed for cancer patients and survivors, including Cancer Wellness for Life, which is an organization that develops oncology exercise resources for individuals, hospitals, and corporations.

There is a LiveFit Cancer Exercise Program[42] offered by the University of North Carolina Healthcare Wellness Centers, which helps cancer survivors ease their way back into physical activity with the help of trained fitness professionals.

Provide your oncologist with a list of programs that interest you and ask for approval to proceed with at least one of those programs.

---

40 "Exercise During Cancer Treatment: An Expert Q&A | Cancer.Net."
41 "The Y: Livestrong® at the YMCA."
42 "LiveFit Cancer Exercise Program - UNC Wellness."

CHAPTER 22:
Food and Diet During Treatment

I truly believed that food could be an excellent complement to my medical treatment and a source of healing. In my search for nutritious food to eat during treatment, I found several websites that had lists of food that would "cure" you if you ate a ton of garlic or pomegranate seeds. Those are all just false schemes to take advantage of those who are desperate for a cure and don't believe they have the right resources available for treatment.

I expressed my concern about healthy eating with my doctor, who did not provide specific advice about nutrition but cautioned me against eating foods with high levels of antioxidants. She drew a picture on a sheet of paper, explaining how they were trying to weaken the cancer cell to attack them, and antioxidants help to create a barrier on the cancer cells and prevent them from being eradicated. I didn't understand the science, but I appreciated her dumbing it down enough, with a drawing, to help me know that I should stay away from eating a whole container of blueberries.

Benefits of healthy eating during treatment

The American Society of Clinical Oncology (ASCO) provides Nutrition Recommendations during and after treatment through their Cancer.Net site. During cancer treatment, I knew I had to maintain a healthy weight, get essential nutrients, and be as active as possible. To get essential nutrients, they recommend visiting with a nutrition counselor. Some cancer centers now offer an in-house nutritionist or Oncology Dietitians for consults with cancer patients.

I was determined to do my part to make healthy food choices to fight this disease. These choices included reducing my soda and sugar intake while increasing my intake of water and organic foods. One of my classic problem areas was my love of carbs.

According to WebMD,[43] what you eat is essential before, during, and after cancer treatment. Before treatment, plan for the upcoming days when side effects may prevent you from focusing on your specific dietary needs. This includes planning, prepping, and storing meals. They suggest, on good days, to eat lots of proteins and healthy calories.

Something I learned the hard way was to drink plenty of fluids. After one chemo treatment, I had an awful side effect, which caused vertigo and vomiting. Both my oncologist and ear doctor suspected it was because of low levels of hydration. They cautioned me to take in plenty of fluids before future treatment sessions.

I experienced many side effects because of treatment, such as nausea, dry mouth, and diarrhea. My oncologist managed some of these side effects with prescription medications, but I was also careful to eat foods that would sustain me during these episodes.

Thankfully, we had a wealth of family members and friends to prepare, cook, and often deliver food. In the beginning, we had more food than we could eat and didn't want it to go to waste, so we ended up managing food delivery with an online tool called LotsaHelpingHands.com. We created a private website that allowed us to select the dates for meals and suggest foods we liked and foods we didn't like.

---

43 "Cancer Diet: Eating Right When You Have Cancer."

We established times when we would like deliveries and were notified when someone signed up. It was beneficial to add notes, such as whether we could entertain guests or preferred the food to be dropped off.

Talking repeatedly about your cancer with family and friends could be very draining, so it was helpful to tell people when conversations needed to take place at a different time. We also had several family members and friends who were far away, send gift cards or ordered meal deliveries. It served as an excellent opportunity for them to take part in my recovery.

Survivor Secret: Nutrition Resources

- The Association of Community Cancer Centers provides a comprehensive listing of Cancer Nutrition Resources on their website (accc-cancer.org/home/learn/patient-centered-care/nutrition/cancer-nutrition-resources), from live and archived events and resources for health professionals to patient education resources.

- The National Cancer Institute provides a comprehensive guide for nutrition called, "Eating Hints: Before, during, and after Cancer Treatment." Many other publications use the guide as a reference. (cancer.gov/publications/patient-education/eatinghints.pdf)

- Mom's Meals offers menu options specifically tailored to meet the nutritional needs of cancer patients. (momsmeals.com/our-food/nutrition/cancer-support/)

- Magnolia Meals at Home ® is a meal delivery program providing nourishing meals at no cost to households affected by cancer. According to their website (magnoliamealsathome.com/), "eligible participants will receive up to two months of home meal deliveries, each of which will include ten meals that are designed to help meet the nutritional needs of cancer patients and up to ten additional meals for their family members if requested by the participant."

- Academy of Nutrition and Dietetics (eatright.org/). Select "Find an Expert"

- Oncology Nutrition Dietetic Practice Group (oncologynutrition.org/)

CHAPTER 23:

Cancer Retreats

Cancer retreats are a rising trend. I took advantage of a retreat when I attended one at a local hospital and was especially impressed. The retreat ran for half a day and focused on health and wellness. Panel members consisted of medical professionals, cancer survivors, and nonprofit and for-profit organizations that provided information on service offerings to cancer survivors.

Sometimes, cancer retreats can become destination-based retreats, such as Casting for Recovery (CfR),[44] which is a free 2 ½- day retreat for women who are going through or have been treated for breast cancer.

A fellow cancer survivor, Marnie, had never heard about them until a relative in another state told her about it. She looked up the program to see if they offered it in our home state of Virginia; it was. After applying for the program, she was selected and very thankful for the opportunity, as this was her first time interacting with other breast cancer survivors away from the constant craziness of breast cancer treatment.

The volunteers welcomed her with compassion, and most were survivors themselves. Throughout the 2 ½- day retreat, there was time for open discussions with certified nurses and psychologists (who are

---

44 cfradmin, "Casting For Recovery | Breast Cancer Fly Fishing Retreats."

volunteers as well), inter-mixed with fly-fishing introductions, practices, and actual fly-fishing (with all the gear needed--including waders).

Here's a "Did you know" fun fact: Fly-fishing casting is one of the gentlest casting techniques to perform. It enables ladies with lymphedema to take part with little to no strain on the arm.

Lisa Esposito, in her article titled "Cancer Retreats: Finding a Fresh Perspective[45]" highlights how survivor getaways offer relaxation, connection, and inspiration in cool locations. And, scientifically, "retreat experiences can lead to substantial improvements in multiple dimensions of health and wellbeing that are maintained for six weeks."[46]

I encourage anyone (survivors, family members, friends) who have been impacted by cancer to consider a retreat. These are amazing experiences that can have a positive impact on your wellbeing.

Survivor Secret: Cancer Retreat Resources

- The Cancer.Net community provides an extensive listing of Cancer Retreats and Camps to include Camp Koru for young survivors, which "is a camp to help cancer survivors diagnosed between the ages of 18-39 to find healing and renewal through outdoor experiences in the ocean and mountains." (cancer.net/navigating-cancer-care/children/camps-and-retreats-families-and-children-affected-cancer)

---

45 Esposito, "Cancer Retreats: Finding a Fresh Perspective."
46 "Do Wellness Tourists Get Well? An Observational Study of Multiple Dimensions of Health and Well-Being After a Week-Long Retreat."

- Mary's Place by the Sea (marysplacebythesea.org/) "provides services that complement their medical treatment, including oncology massage, nutrition education, individual counseling, Reiki, guided meditation, expressive writing, and yoga. They offer integrative services to women with cancer and provide rest and support during this challenging time in their lives. Before they leave, they are empowered with knowledge that will aid them on their road to healing."

Part 6

WHAT NORMAL LOOKS LIKE NOW

CHAPTER 24:

Returning to Normalcy

I was so glad when I could finally ring the bell, signifying the completion of over 30 rounds of radiation treatments. It was a special moment I shared with my husband, and it marked the end of a long eight months of active cancer treatment. I completed three phases of treatment: chemotherapy, surgery (double mastectomy), and radiation.

Although I was thrilled to have made it this far, I was reluctant to have a huge celebration to mark the conclusion of this journey because, with IBC, I knew there was a high risk of cancer recurrence. I would have to be continuously monitored. They expected to see me at least twice a year for the next five years and then once a year after that. In my opinion, their definition of continuous monitoring did not meet my expectations.

When I finished treatment and had no more appointments to attend, I felt a kind of loss. Were they sure I was okay? How did they know? Could I be tested every month? Wait for what? I have to wait for six months to conduct my next series of tests to detect cancer. How ludicrous! What if it comes back within those six months? How will I know if I'm not getting scanned every month? They said this type of cancer was aggressive! They call this scanxiety, and it's common for cancer patients – it's a build-up of anxiety because of the fear the cancer may return, and that following a scan, you'll hear the dreaded words again, "you have cancer."

I expected to see them at least once a month. I had just completed radiation where I would see the nurses every weekday and the radiation oncologist once a week.

Before that, I had a regular rotation of visits with the hematology oncologist interspersed with visits with the surgeon. To go from daily and/or weekly visits to only seeing a doctor once every 6-months was rather frightening. I had found comfort in being seen regularly.

There was a team of doctors, nurses, and caregivers surrounding me every week, and having them there assured me progress was being made, and I would be okay. Then suddenly, nothing. Treatment is over, they're gone, and doubts crept back into my mind. Any time something felt abnormal, or I had any pain, it had to be examined. One time, I was driving home, and I felt a pain in my chest that wouldn't go away. I called my husband to tell him what was going on and that I was going to the hospital to get checked out.

I commend the emergency room doctors for taking me seriously and doing the full workup with testing and everything. It turns out it was pain from the surgery that was months past. The scar tissue underneath the surface was still contracting, and that was the pain I was feeling.

I felt stupid, causing all this commotion, but my oncologist assured me it was normal and good for me to keep a close eye on my body. She told me not to be afraid to ask questions or ask for help when I needed it. If there was a recurrence, both she and I wanted to address it as soon as possible.

To cope, I would do my best to push the thoughts of it out of my mind as much as possible and occupy my mind with work and family. It was difficult because the result of the cancer screenings would determine whether I could proceed with my next stage of treatment. This included surgery to reduce the likelihood of recurrence and reconstruction surgery. In conducting research into this unmet need for cancer survivors, caregivers, and friends, I came across Alexia Holovatyk, M.S., Ph.D. Candidate, who received psycho-oncology training at the UCLA Simms/Mann Center for Integrative Oncology.

Alexia is passionate about providing much-needed psychosocial support to cancer survivors, and in her experience, the most significant unmet need for cancer survivors is knowing how to cope with the fear of cancer recurrence. She's heard so many people say, "I know I could get hit by a car anytime, but living with the risk that the cancer might come back is especially tough." While everyone "knows" they might die at any time, this fact is especially salient for survivors of cancer, and they can't "unknow" this vulnerability.

Marie Ennis O'Connor provides some practical advice for coping with scanxiety, some of which include breaking the worry habit and creating an anxiety worry period. She shares that since worrying is a habit, we can break habits. By creating a worry period, you acknowledge the worry, but don't let it control your life.[47]

Rehabilitation

Luckily for me, my cancer surgeon made sure I had access to a cancer rehabilitation doctor. I met with this doctor during chemotherapy and had follow-up appointments with him post-surgery.

The visit before surgery was an opportunity to meet the doctor and discuss my current treatment plan and gain an understanding of the side effects. They could also get a baseline of my health via a questionnaire, follow-up questions, and some minor testing.

Because I was being treated for breast cancer, the doctor already knew many of the side effects that I was experiencing and provided some recommendations to counter them. He also knew there would be

---

47 Ennis-O'Connor, "Coping with Scanxiety: Practical Tips from Cancer Patients."

some longer-lasting side effects following treatment. There are two specific side effects I will share: one, Frozen Shoulder, and the other, lymphedema.

Frozen Shoulder is a condition where there is a stiffness in the shoulder joint that can limit the rotation of the ball and socket joint. Sometimes, it can be painful. Before my surgery, the rehabilitation doctor collaborated with my surgeon to provide a course of treatment for physical therapy for both the Frozen Shoulder and lymphedema.

The rehab doctor recommended a physical therapist who specialized in lymphedema treatment and prevention that I should visit following recovery from surgery.

Because of the operation, I could no longer have blood drawn or blood pressure checks administered on the same arm that had lymph nodes removed as this could risk infection and an onslaught of lymphedema.

The rehab doctor also shared that some side effects, such as neuropathy in my fingers and feet, would subside. The feeling in my fingers returned to normal much more quickly than my feet. It was a matter of weeks for my fingers, but months for my feet to return to normal feeling. Seeing the physical therapist and lymphedema therapist helped with the healing process and returning to normal.

Back to Being Mom/Dad, Husband/Wife, Family Member, Friend

Alexia Holovatyk says that another big challenge is navigating back into everyday life and back into roles, such as "mom/dad," husband/wife," and "friend." The expectation is that once cancer treatment is over, the person can simply "return to their normal life." The reality is that a person may need to redefine how they engage with those roles, and it probably won't look the same.

An additional challenge a survivor may have is talking about difficulties with sexual functioning and intimacy after a diagnosis/ treatment. Unfortunately, many doctors still don't have a great deal of expertise in this area, but help exists, and it's essential for people to feel comfortable enough to have these discussions.

There are some barriers to getting help post-treatment. For one thing, people may not think it is "normal" to need support after completing treatment (shouldn't they be happy they beat cancer?). A massive win would have oncologists inform people that it is very typical and expected that people who just went through a cancer diagnosis would benefit from psychosocial support.

Returning to Work After Cancer

The cancer treatments were very taxing and left me unable to work. But as the treatment cycle was ending, I thought about returning to work.

I received a call from a former coworker who was checking in on me and wanted to know my level of interest in returning to work. I expressed some reluctance to return because I was recovering from surgery and about to begin radiation treatment, which causes a great deal of fatigue.

My colleague asked if it would be of interest to me in returning to work in a part-time status that could accommodate my remaining treatment regimen? I let him know it sounded appealing and to let me know if such an opportunity became available.

A few weeks later, he called and said there was an opportunity for me to work on a contract part-time, and the hours were flexible to accommodate my treatment schedule. I agreed to proceed with the plan and readied myself to return to work.

I knew it would be both mentally and physically demanding to return to work. Besides working on-site, I would return to a 35-mile commute each way. Thankfully, I could plan out my radiation treatments to occur in the afternoons, and the treatment center was close to my home. The fatigue would not affect my short commute from the radiation treatment center to my house.

I had to prepare myself to return to work mentally. I was bald, and my eyebrows and eyelashes were just beginning to return. I was used to wearing headscarves and wigs since the early stages of chemotherapy, but there was still a bit of reluctance to return to the office with no hair. I swallowed my pride and returned to work.

In addition to me returning to normalcy, my husband was undergoing the same transition.

Words from a Caregiver: Husband (Keith)

"The return to normalcy wasn't so bad, but a full return to life as we knew it would take a little longer than we originally planned. Cancer treatments greatly impact your immune system, so the one thing we didn't want to do was rush her back to work. As a matter of fact, we didn't even know what that should look like. Should she go part-time, should she even go back to work?

The toll of cancer doesn't just impact the person diagnosed, but it takes a massive toll on the caregiver. I was stressed, tired, and I needed some time just to get away and decompress. My biggest fear was being able to maintain the lifestyle that we had if she didn't return to work. I didn't want to uproot my family from the only life they knew, so selfishly, I wanted her to return to work.

My best friend called and said he was taking a trip to the Caribbean and asked if I could join him. I didn't know how that would be taken, but I decided to do just that; I needed to get away from the frenzied and hectic lifestyle that I had. Selfish, maybe, but you only get one life. You have to take care of yourself every now and then. Initially, my wife wasn't happy about me taking this trip, but she understood. Over the course of that year, the only thing that mattered was my wife, her health, and doing what I needed to do for our children. During that time, I had not taken care of myself, and that needed some attention.

Once I arrived at my destination, I slept for the first few days. If I wasn't sleeping, I was outside on the patio, watching and listening to the ocean and enjoying the ocean breeze. The rhythmic sound of the waves crashing on the beach was soothing; it took me away, away from everything that I was living and everything that I feared. When I returned, I was ready for whatever was next; my stress was gone, and my mental battery had been recharged.

My biggest takeaway is that you cannot be of assistance to anyone that needs you if you are not in a position to assist. If you are not healthy, then whatever you can do will be limited. Life throws enough stress at you; add in a debilitating disease to someone you love and need, and your stress levels can go through the roof. Take time to breathe, take time for yourself, be selfish, even if it's just for a little while."

Survivor Secret: Resources for Returning to Normalcy

- Many Cancer Support Communities provide free individual support to cancer survivors. cancersupportcommunity.org/

- Sharsheret is an organization that provides psychosocial support over the phone to women who have had breast or ovarian cancer (sharsheret.org/)

- An article with useful tips if you are striving to have a positive attitude with cancer: (verywellhealth.com/ how-to-keep-a-positive-attitude-with-cancer-2248819)

- Helpful tips for returning to work are available from Cancer and Careers (cancerandcareers.org/). The mission of Cancer and Careers is to empower and educate people with cancer to thrive in their workplace by providing expert advice, interactive tools, and educational events.

- The American Cancer Society offers some additional considerations for returning to work after cancer treatment, including telling coworkers about treatment, your legal protections as a cancer survivor, reasonable accommodations, and the potential for workplace discrimination. More details can be found on their website:(cancer.org/treatment/finding-and-paying-for-treatment/understanding-financial-and-legal-matters/ working-during-and-after-treatment/returning-to-work-after-cancer-treatment.html).

CHAPTER 25:
Winning the Battle

Words from a Caregiver: Husband (Keith)

"The battle was long, hard and arduous. Through the pain and tears, the destination that seemed unreachable and unattainable had been reached. My wife rang The Final Bell that signified the end of her radiation treatment and the end of her cancer treatment. I remember the look on my wife's face; she had a smile that couldn't be contained. I kissed her, and to this day, I don't know how I held back the stream of tears that were building. I remember the nurses all gathering in the halls, cheering her on, and she took the final steps towards a healthy future.

We got home, cried and reminisced on the journey. What if we didn't have, as the doctor said, rock star insurance or any insurance for that matter? Would the outcome have been the same, would 'we' be sitting here today? It was at this point that my wife felt a nudge of God's presence; she knew what she was going to do with her life. She would help the people who were unable to help themselves; her journey was a testimony of God's grace in her life. He put her through it so that she could be able to speak to it firsthand.

As for me, I had my wife. Nothing much has changed; we argue, fuss and fight like everyone else. The blessing is, she is still here. She is my reason. She is the one that completes me. Everything that I have attained, she has been a part of it. I don't know what I would be or where I would be without her. Although the physical battle was hers, I fought with her all the way, and because of God's grace, my wife gets to spend every day with me and our children. I remember that call to my father in law, telling him that his daughter's journey was complete. I no longer felt broken; with her journey complete, I felt whole, my promise realized.

So, for those of you going through your own ordeal, what would I say to you? I would say, be thankful. You were chosen because of your strength; you are the light that someone else will need to successfully combat cancer or some other medical condition. Someone is watching you; show grace, be vulnerable, and when it is all done, smile and be grateful."

****

I started my cancer journey on January 25, 2013. Although I have received a clean bill of health after the conclusion of treatments in November of the same year, my journey continues. The impact cancer has had on my life has been tremendous. I have had so many emotions in dealing with this disease: fear, anger, anxiety, loneliness, strength. It is through my battle with this disease that I uncovered my calling.

I believe we all have a calling. Sometimes, when we are in search of that calling, we are met with a challenge that might seem impossible. IBC was my challenge. I faced it head-on and beat it at its own game. Because of that battle, I know my calling is to help people deal with this dreadful disease called cancer.

I am a cancer advocate. My story may be like yours or entirely different; however, we are the same. We are SURVIVORS! Cancer will always be a part of our life journey. We embrace it and make the choice to live life to the fullest and on purpose. As long as we do that, cancer will not win.

Acknowledgments

I must start by thanking God for His grace and healing powers. Thank you to my wonderful husband, Keith. He has loved and supported me throughout this cancer journey and has shown in many ways the true meaning of "in sickness and in health."

A few years after treatment, I shared with Keith how I realized that my purpose in life was to help cancer patients and survivors get access to the information they need to survive this dreadful disease. He listened and encouraged me to take the steps necessary to fulfill this purpose. Sincerely, I thank you and love you.

To my Mom and Dad, Patricia and Frank McClain, who kept me encouraged and continuously lifted up in prayer. Thank you for the many nights you listened as I vented my fears and frustrations. In return, I received your unyielding support and motivation. Please know you are much appreciated, and no one can ever take your place.

To my sweet, sweet babies, Kelci, Kendall, and Keith Jr., who are all so resilient and wise beyond their years. From my diagnosis and when I was in the battle, my love for you kept me going. It was in my thoughts that I uncovered a strength that I never knew I had. I love you all so much.

To my sister, Delisa Pettus, and brother, Aaron McClain, I thank you for your love and for keeping me laughing through it all and listening to my many ideas.

To my mother-in-law and father-in-law, Brenda and Joe Nolen, thank you for your love and support and for being a sounding board for your son.

To my Aunt Elaine, thank you for coming to take care of us and your loving spirit.

I thank my cancer team of oncologists and surgeons who cared for me throughout this journey: Dr. Amy Irwin, Dr. Stella Hetelekidis, Dr. Massimo Cristofanilli, Dr. Mark Boisvert, and Dr. Christopher Trahan. I pushed each of you extremely hard, and you all accepted the challenge.

To all the fantastic cancer patients and survivors I met along the way, I thank you for sharing your heart and words of wisdom. A special thank you to survivor contributors who I met along the way and contributed their stories, including Marnie, Dara, Tanja, and Austyn.

Thank you to Alexia Holovatyk who answered my online questions and for her contributions to this book.

A special thank you to a local survivor, Liz Tobin, who took me under her wings and introduced me to the amazing Terry Arnold, founder of The IBC Network Foundation. The work by this nonprofit organization and the research it funds is helping to save lives like mine.

Thanks to Linda Griffin, of Grassroots Marketing Systems, LLC., who has helped me take the idea of a book to reality. There were many starts and stops, but she was persistent in ensuring we made it to the finish line.

Thank you to my extended family members, friends, church family, and Delta Sigma Theta Sorors who have prayed, brought food, helped care for our children, or just listened. I will not forget your gestures.

Bibliography

Cancer Support Community | Cancer Support Community. "A to Z List of Cancer Support Resources | Cancer Support Community." Accessed July 2, 2020. https://www.cancersupportcommunity.org/resources.

Attorney, Amy Loftsgordon. "What's the Difference Between PMI and Mortgage Protection Insurance? | Nolo." www.nolo.com. Nolo, October 28, 2013. http://nolo.com/legal-encyclopedia/whats-the-difference-between-pmi-mortgage-protection-insurance.html.

SHARE Cancer Support. "Breast & Ovarian Cancer Charity | SHARE Cancer Support." Accessed July 2, 2020. https://www.sharecancersupport.org/.

Breast Cancer Foundation | Susan G. Komen®. "Breast Cancer Prescription Drug Assistance | Susan G. Komen®." Accessed July 2, 2020. http://ww5.komen.org/BreastCancer/PrescriptionDrugs.html.

Brock, Melissa. "Cancer Costs: Resources To Manage Housing Expenses During Treatment | Bankrate." Bankrate. Bankrate.com, January 27, 2020. https://www.bankrate.com/mortgages/how-to-afford-home-expenses-during-cancer-treatment/.

Amazon.com: Online Shopping for Electronics, Apparel, Computers, Books, DVDs & more. "Cancer ... and I: A 365 Day Guided Diary to Journal Your Cancer Emotions: Grobler, Ronell: 9781518619199:

Amazon.Com: Books." Accessed July 2, 2020. http://amazon.com/Cancer-Guided-Diary-Journal-Emotions/dp/1518619193/ref=sr_1_3?keywords=guided+journaling+cancer&qid=1583937834&s=books&sr=1-3.

Bibliography

WebMD. "Cancer Diet: Eating Right When You Have Cancer." WebMD, 9AD. http://webmd.com/cancer/cancer-diet#.

CancerQuest. "Cancer Disparities | CancerQuest." Accessed July 2, 2020. http://cancerquest.org/patients/cancer-disparities.

National Cancer Institute. "Cancer Disparities - National Cancer Institute." Accessed July 2, 2020. http://cancer.gov/about-cancer/understanding/disparities.

American Cancer Society | Information and Resources about for Cancer: Breast, Colon, Lung, Prostate, Skin. "Cancer Facts & Figures 2016 | American Cancer Society." Accessed July 2, 2020. http://cancer.org/research/cancer-facts-statistics/all-cancer-facts-figures/cancer-facts-figures-2016.html.

PubMed Central (PMC). "Cancer Patient Navigator Tasks across the Cancer Care Continuum." Accessed July 2, 2020. http://ncbi.nlm.nih.gov/pmc/articles/PMC3302357/.

Medscape. "Cancer Patients Report Lack of Info and Support," 8AD. https://www.medscape.com/viewarticle/916361.

NCCS - National Coalition for Cancer Survivorship. "Cancer Survival Toolbox." https://www.facebook.com/cancersurvivorship/. Accessed July 2, 2020. http://canceradvocacy.org/resources/cancer-survival-toolbox/.

Centers for Disease Control and Prevention. "CDC: 1 in 4 US Adults Live with a Disability | CDC Online Newsroom | CDC." Accessed July 2, 2020. https://www.cdc.gov/media/releases/2018/p0816-disability.html.

cfradmin. "Casting For Recovery | Breast Cancer Fly Fishing Retreats." Casting for Recovery. Casting for Recovery. Accessed July 2, 2020. http://castingforrecovery.org/.

ch. "Guided Journaling — Collaboratio Helvetica." collaboratio helvetica. collaboratio helvetica, February 27, 2019. http://collaboratiohelvetica.ch/blog/2019/02/05/send-a-30-sc6dl.

Chang, Ellen. "Mortgage Protection Insurance: When You Might Need It | Bankrate." Bankrate. Bankrate.com, January 30, 2020. https://www.bankrate.com/mortgages/do-you-need-mortgage-protection-insurance/.

Bibliography

Patient Power. "Communicating Cancer to Adult Children | Patient Power." Accessed July 2, 2020. http://patientpower.info/navigating-cancer/care-partners/ communicating-cancer-to-adult-children.

PubMed Central (PMC). "Do Wellness Tourists Get Well? An Observational Study of Multiple Dimensions of Health and Well-Being After a Week-Long Retreat." Accessed July 2, 2020. http://ncbi.nlm.nih.gov/pmc/articles/PMC5312624/.

Eldridge, Lynn. "How to Advocate for Yourself as a Cancer Patient." Verywell Health. Accessed July 2, 2020. https://www.verywellhealth.com/how-to-be-your-own-advocate-as-a-cancer-patient-2248881.

Ennis-O'Connor, Marie. "Coping with Scanxiety: Practical Tips from Cancer Patients." Powerful Patients, July 24, 2018. powerfulpatients.org.

Esposito, Lisa. "Cancer Retreats: Finding a Fresh Perspective." usnews.com, June 3, 2015. https://health.usnews.com/health-news/patient-advice/articles/2015/06/03/ cancer-retreats-finding-a-fresh-perspective.

Cancer.Net. "Exercise During Cancer Treatment: An Expert Q&A | Cancer.Net," May 11, 2017. http://cancer.net/blog/2017-05/exercise-during-cancer-treatment-expert-qa.

Official web site of the U.S. Health Resources & Services Administration. "Federally Qualified Health Centers | Official Web Site of the U.S. Health Resources & Services Administration," April 21, 2017. https://www.hrsa.gov/opa/eligibility-and-registration/health-centers/fqhc/index.html#:~:text=Federally%20Qualified%20 Health%20Centers%20are,care%20services%20in%20underserved%20areas.

Fellow, Crystal McCown - Social Work Counselor. "Journaling Your Way through Cancer | MD Anderson Cancer Center." MD Anderson Cancer Center. MD Anderson Cancer Center, April 9, 2013. http://mdanderson.org/publications/ cancerwise/practicing-self-care-through-journaling.h00-158828856.html.

Forster, Victoria. "Why Do Only Eight Percent Of Cancer Patients In The U.S. Participate In Clinical Trials?" Forbes. Forbes, February 19, 2019. http://forbes.com/ sites/victoriaforster/2019/02/19/why-do-only-eight-percent-of-cancer-patients-in-the-u-s-participate-in-clinical-trials/#5567d12777e9.

CancerCare. "Free Resource for People with Cancer." Accessed July 2, 2020. http://cancerfac.org.

American Cancer Society | Information and Resources about for Cancer: Breast, Colon, Lung, Prostate, Skin. "How Do I Find a Clinical Trial That's Right for Me?" Accessed July 2, 2020. http://cancer.org/treatment/treatments-and-side-effects/clinical-trials/what-you-need-to-know/picking-a-clinical-trial.html.

Amazon.com: Online Shopping for Electronics, Apparel, Computers, Books, DVDs & more. "Journaling Through Breast Cancer: Bergsma, Christine: 9780986965531: Amazon.Com: Books." Accessed July 2, 2020. http://amazon.com/gp/product/0986965537/ref=dbs_a_def_rwt_bibl_vppi_i0.

Known, Cancer Caregivers - Things I Wish I'd. "Cancer Caregivers - Things I Wish I'd Known - Resources." Cancer Caregivers - Things I Wish I'd Known - Home. Accessed July 2, 2020. http://thingsiwishidknown.com/index.php?pageID=11244.

UNC Wellness. "LiveFit Cancer Exercise Program - UNC Wellness." Accessed July 2, 2020. https://uncwellness.com/services/livefit-cancer-exercise-program/.

Press Room | Career Builder. "Living Paycheck to Paycheck Is a Way of Life for Majority of U.S. Workers, According to New CareerBuilder Survey - Aug 24, 2017." Accessed July 2, 2020. http://press.careerbuilder.com/2017-08-24-Living-Paycheck-to-Paycheck-is-a-Way-of-Life-for-Majority-of-U-S-Workers-According-to-New-CareerBuilder-Survey.

Monique. "Exercise as Part of Cancer Treatment - Harvard Health Blog - Harvard Health Publishing." Harvard Health Blog, June 13, 2018. https://www.health.harvard.edu/blog/exercise-as-part-of-cancer-treatment-2018061314035.

NCCC | home. "NCCC | Home." Accessed July 2, 2020. http://nccc.georgetown.edu/index.php.

One-on-one support for adults impacted by cancer. "One-on-One Support for Adults Impacted by Cancer." Accessed July 2, 2020. http://cancerhopenetwork.org.

Choose Hope. "Our Top 5 Cancer Gift Ideas for Chemo Patients | Choose Hope," September 16, 2019. http://choosehope.com/blog/top-5-cancer-gift-ideas-chemo-patients/.

Bibliography

American Cancer Society | Information and Resources about for Cancer: Breast, Colon, Lung, Prostate, Skin. "Road To Recovery." Accessed July 2, 2020. http://cancer.org/treatment/support-programs-and-services/road-to-recovery.html.

Robbins, Mike. "It's OK to Ask for Help | HuffPost Life." HuffPost. HuffPost, January 29, 2011. https://m.huffpost.com/us/entry/814796.

Sasson, Remez. "How Many Thoughts Does Your Mind Think in One Hour?" Success Consciousness - Skills for Success, Positivity and Inner Peace. Accessed July 2, 2020. http://successconsciousness.com/blog/inner-peace/how-many-thoughts-does-your-mind-think-in-one-hour/.

Lotsa Helping Hands. "Staying Positive and Making Chemotherapy Hair Loss Look Good," May 28, 2015. http://lotsahelpinghands.com/blog/chemotherapy-hair-loss/.

Cancer.Net. "Support Groups | Cancer.Net," December 18, 2009. http://cancer.net/coping-with-cancer/finding-support-and-information/support-groups.

the Y. "The Y : Livestrong® at the YMCA." https://www.facebook.com/ymca, April 28, 2017. http://ymca.net/livestrong-at-the-ymca.

Verma, Prakhar. "Destroy Negativity From Your Mind With This Simple Exercise." Medium. Mission.org, November 27, 2017. http://medium.com/the-mission/a-practical-hack-to-combat-negative-thoughts-in-2-minutes-or-less-cc3d1bddb3af.

Think Cultural Health. "What Is CLAS? - Think Cultural Health." Accessed July 2, 2020. http://thinkculturalhealth.hhs.gov/clas/what-is-clas.

Accessed July 2, 2020. https://ascopubs.org/doi/10.1200/JCO.2006.06.5300.

Accessed July 2, 2020. https://app.emergingmed.com/emed/home.

Made in United States
Orlando, FL
26 October 2022

23875643R00093